RESTFUL

SLEEP

DEEPAK CHOPRA, M.D.

RESTFUL

SLEEP

the complete mind/body

program for overcoming

insomnia

 THREE RIVERS PRESS • NEW YORK

Published by Three Rivers Press, New York, New York.
Member of the Crown Publishing Group.

Originally published in hardcover by Harmony Books in 1994.

Random House, Inc. New York, Toronto, London, Sydney, Auckland.
www.randomhouse.com

Portions of this book were originally published on audiocassette by
Quantum Publications as part of the Perfect Health Series in 1991.

THREE RIVERS PRESS is a registered trademark and the Three Rivers Press
colophon is a trademark of Random House, Inc.

Printed in the United States of America

Library of Congress Cataloging-in-Publication Data

Chopra, Deepak.
  Restful sleep : The complete mind/body program for overcoming
insomnia / Deepak Chopra.
       p.   cm.
  1. Insomnia—Treatment.   2. Insomnia—Popular works.   3. Medicine,
Ayurvedic.   I. Title
RC548.C47   1994
616.8'498—dc20
94-19244
CIP

ISBN 0-517-88457-7

10   9   8

CONTENTS

RESTFUL
SLEEP

Sleep and the

Quantum

Mechanical Body

Sleep, like good health in general, is something most people take for granted. As long as it's coming easily, there's just no reason to give it much thought. But for millions of people, a good night's sleep isn't easily come by—and as you'll learn throughout this book, the reasons for that are more far-reaching and more complex than you might suspect.

Is insomnia more prevalent in our society today, as millions of us lie awake at night, worrying, mentally balancing our checkbooks, replaying arguments and misunderstandings until there's finally nothing left to do but get up and watch television?

At present this is certainly a nation of troubled sleepers. Based on the number of prescriptions written for sleeping pills and the volume of commercially produced sleep aids, insomnia may be our most widespread health problem. Virtually everyone has experienced insomnia occasionally, and currently one out of every three adults experience periodic trouble with sleeping. Each year, at least 10 million Americans consult physicians about their sleep, and about half of them receive prescriptions for sleeping pills. A survey by the National Institutes of Health conducted in the 1970s revealed that 17 percent of the total population was bothered greatly by insomnia, and among older people the percentage was even higher, with one out of every four people over the age of 60 reporting serious sleep difficulties. And when sleep difficulties arise, the basic human function that we may have once taken for granted is transformed into a labyrinth of anxiety.

Chances are good that right now you're surrounded by sleepy people. They're everywhere, many of them driving cars or operating sensitive equipment. They seem unable to get a good night's sleep; or, even if they do, they're convinced that they *don't*, so the effect is the same, at least psychologically. Many of these people are elderly, but a significant percentage is young. There's a perception that older people need less sleep—that insomnia among the elderly is to be taken for granted—but that's only because older people's sleeplessness is so widespread, not because it's a natural condition. Similarly, college students might seem a relatively carefree group who simply choose to stay up late. But in fact the biological need for sleep is greater between the ages of 17 and 25 than at any time since infancy. So, if young people are sleep-deprived, it's likely due to social or academic pressures.

Both young adults and the elderly consume significant amounts of alcohol. When a chronically sleepless person takes a drink, the effect is multiplied, so that a single beer can be as debilitating as a six-pack, according to sleep researchers.

I don't know anyone who hasn't experienced insomnia at one time or another, and I've had a number of patients who were serious problem sleepers. I'm glad to report that I also don't know anyone who hasn't experienced major benefits from the techniques presented in this book. Some of these ideas are derived from Ayurveda, the traditional medicine of India; others are the result of Western scientific research. Most significant, you can expect improvement right away, even if you haven't had a good night's sleep in years.

Before we begin to learn these techniques, I'd like to suggest an insight that was given to me by a woman who had been deeply troubled by chronic insomnia. I think it will be very useful, not only for its practical specifics but because it suggests one of the fundamental ideas that runs through this book: That is, what happens to you at night when you try to sleep cannot be understood except in terms of what you do during the day, when you're awake.

For years my patient had lain awake trying to sleep. Then, very late one night, she had an important realization about the source of her insomnia: There were *things left undone* in her waking life that made her, unconsciously, uncomfortable with going to sleep. There were active, positive things that she wanted to do, and until she did them she simply wasn't ready to sleep. These unsatisfied aspirations—such as traveling, writing, or getting back in touch with old friends—weren't things she could simply jump out of bed and take care of on the night she had this realization. Rather, they required a long-term re-orienting of her life. Once she began that process, her sleep improved because her waking life had improved. The goal of this book is to help you do *both* those things in your life.

SLEEP: WHAT IT IS AND WHAT IT ISN'T

Sleep is a distinct state of mind and body in which the body is deeply at rest, the metabolism is lowered, and the mind becomes unconscious to the outside world. This last phrase must be examined carefully, for we all know that the sleeping mind does not become unconscious entirely; instead, it shifts the direction of consciousness from, say, a chair beside your bed to another chair inside your dream. In fact, in terms of its biological functions, the brain is really "working harder" during the dreaming period of sleep than it is during the day. Moreover, within that reoriented but not completely "resting" state, there are further gradations that vary from one individual to another and from one part of the sleep cycle to another. Just as some people seem more awake than others during the day, so some people are "more asleep" during the night.

However, with respect to *good sleep*, the elusive goal for which so many are striving, I think there are some general statements that can help us to recognize the phenomenon, if not exactly to define it:

- Good quality sleep seems to happen by itself. You don't have to fight for it against restlessness or anxiety, and you don't have to take drugs of any kind to experience it.
- You rarely wake up in the middle of the night from good sleep, but if you do, you get back to sleep quickly without worrying about it.
- You wake up naturally in the morning. You're neither sluggish and groggy nor anxious and hyperalert.
- Finally, good sleep provides you with a sense of vitality that lasts throughout the day. You don't feel you've been deprived of rest during the preceding night, and you don't feel anxious about what's going to happen the next time you try to fall asleep.

These are some subjective characteristics of sleep from the sleeper's point of view. It's also useful, here at the outset, to look at the more detached observations about sleep that have emerged from clinical studies.

When researchers study human physiological characteristics over a twenty-four-hour period, including measurements of the brain waves known as electroencephalography, or EEG, they find that four distinct states of consciousness, or psychophysiology, emerge. These are:

- Deep sleep, or delta sleep, during which most rest and restoration takes place
- The dream state, also known as REM sleep because of the rapid eye movements that accompany it
- Light sleep, which often takes up a majority of the time during the night, and which occurs after the above two periods have ended
- The waking state, in which you find yourself as you read this book

During each twenty-four-hour period, these four states tend to alternate within each individual according to certain regular progressions or rhythms.

Problems with sleep crop up at different points in the daily sequence. Some people have difficulty in falling asleep. Others awaken during the night, sometimes frequently, and have trouble falling asleep again. Still others awaken in the early hours, at about 3:00 or 4:00 A.M., and cannot fall back to sleep. Of course, a combination of these different sleep problems can occur.

Why do we fall asleep in the first place? What's the purpose of sleep? This is a mystery of very long standing. Aristotle proposed that the purpose of sleep was to help the body digest food—although eating a big meal before getting into bed is one of the worst things you can do for your rest. Today sleep is a closely studied biological phenomenon, but scientists are still not in agreement about some of its most fundamental aspects. Some have even proposed that sleep has *no* purely biological function but is simply a coping mechanism left over from prehistoric times, designed to force the primitive human organism to seek safe shelter during the dangerous period of darkness. This adaptive behavior would have the additional benefit of preserving caloric energy that would otherwise have been expended during the cold hours of the night. According to this theory, every night of sleep is like a mini-hibernation.

In my view, the purpose of sleep is to allow the body to repair and rejuvenate itself. The deep rest provided during sleep allows the body to recover from fatigue and stress and enlivens the body's own self-repair and homeostatic, or balancing, mechanisms. Dreaming seems to be a further elaboration of this process of purifying and cleansing stress and tension from the nervous system. Studies on sleep and dream deprivation support these theories.

It's common knowledge that being deprived of a good night's sleep leads to a diminished sense of well-being the next day. We don't feel that we can function at our peak, and we feel more vulnerable to the effects of stress, both mental and physical. In actual fact, however, one sleepless night has virtually no measurable effect on our ability to carry out normal responsibilities the following day, and this has been demonstrated in dozens of studies. In 1964, as part of an experiment for a high school science fair, a California student stayed awake for eleven days and was still able to function reasonably well on the last day. At the conclusion of the experiment he slept for fifteen hours and suffered no short-term or long-term ill effects.

Nevertheless, the perception of fatigue and impaired ability is there, so it is important that we learn how to gain the most deep and refreshing rest from our sleep. This will bring maximum vitality and rejuvenation to both mind and body.

CONSCIOUSNESS AND THE QUANTUM MECHANICAL BODY

To accomplish restful sleep, we need to understand more about the nature of the mind and the body, the connection between them, and the cycles of nature that are so intimately related to our sleep patterns. At this point I would like to introduce you to the concept of the quantum mechanical body/mind, and its connection to the most basic tenents of Ayurveda, the ancient tradition of Indian medicine on which this book is based.

One of the most basic premises of Ayurveda is that the body is a projection of one's consciousness.

Consciousness is another one of those fundamental biological occurrences that is easier to recognize than to define. I think of consciousness as a field of awareness, a field of intelligence. Intelligence alone is nothing more than fields of self-referring information. Let me explain. When a system has a feedback loop that allows it to influence its own expression—as the thermostat of a home heating system can influence the furnace down in the basement—then it acquires a new property. That property is information that is self-correcting. Biological systems have the ability to influence their own expression from moment to moment. Although we cannot call a heating system intelligent, because it is based on a mechanical feedback loop, a heating system with a thermostat provides a model for how the body's intelligence or awareness operates.

Your body is a field of living information, with feedback loops constantly in place. And this living information is also what we can call a field of infinite correlation, which means it can do an infinite number of things all at the same time and coordinate those activities with each other. A human body can kill germs and play a piano and digest food and eliminate toxins and think a philosophy and make a baby all at the same time.

That's only the beginning. The human body doesn't exist in isolation, but part of a larger field of living information that we call Earth. And Earth is then a part of the still larger field of information that comprises the universe. Nature is a continuum in which we cannot separate the human body from the cosmic body, although we are conditioned by our perceptions to do so every day.

We perceive our physical selves as tangible objects only because of the limits of our viewpoint. The seemingly irrefutable reality of the body is, if not exactly an illusion, at least a very limited version of what's really happening.

In truth, the body is constantly remaking itself—literally creating and destroying itself—in every second of its existence. The human body completely renews itself amazingly often: 98 percent of all the cells that make up the human body are new in one year. Every year your physical body is completely different from the one that you had a year ago. It's completely renewed, completely changed at the cellular level.

All this means that today's physical body is quite different from yesterday's—because every six weeks you make a new liver, every month you make a new layer of skin, every five days you make a new stomach lining, and even your skeleton is renewed every three months. So the fact is that the human body is like a river that's constantly flowing, constantly *in process* itself in every second of its existence.

Just as every river must have a source, this river of molecules or atoms is actually a result of vibrations in a field of energy. The energy fields become the molecules of the body. For example, if you look at the atom, the basic unit of matter, you'll see that it is made up of several elementary particles that are whizzing around at incredible speeds through huge, empty spaces. These particles appear to emerge from a field that is completely void: they appear, they rebound, they collide, and then they seem to disappear back into the void. They're there for just a moment. And when we freeze them in a moment of attention, then they give us the appearance of matter, but in fact they are simply fluctuations of energy and information.

Both matter and energy are expressions of a deeper reality. This deeper reality is a field that contains all possible states of matter, information, and energy in the form of pure potentiality. In other words, they are *unmanifest*. They are only there as possibilities, which have yet to differentiate and ultimately express themselves in any measurable form. So behind the mask of your physical body is a quantum mechanical body. This derives from an underlying source that orchestrates, in a very orderly fashion, the fluctuations of energy and information that formally manifest themselves as your physical body.

When you begin to think of the body in this way, the idea that it's a fixed, immutable object seems not only wrong but extremely limiting. Then, the quantum mechanical body emerges as consisting of patterns of intelligence, fields of information, living information that we call intelligence.

Although we think of thoughts, feelings, emotions, and desires as being nonmaterial and the body as being material, both are expressions of the same field of intelligence. A wave of energy, when it is caught in a moment of attention, appears as a particle. But it is a wave at the same time. And the wave is just a fluctuation in the larger field, also at the same time. So whether we see a certain event in the body as a material event, as a mental event, or as just a fluctuation in the field, it's just a matter of our own perspective.

It's important to look closely at all this because these ideas are the foundation on which the modern Ayurvedic approach to health is built—including the sleep-related techniques you'll learn in this book. Einstein (who usually slept about ten hours a night) once said that instead of being a model for actual space/time events, a field is the continuum of possible information states. It's an environment that contains within itself all possible events, as a function of time.

In other words, a field is not a space/time event by itself; a field is a continuum of all possible energy and information states that can then manifest themselves as space/time events. And what do we call these events? We call them tables and chairs, or rocks and trees. We call them *matter*, and that includes the physical body. But in fact that too is just a matter of perspective. All these events are part of a continuum.

Recent scientific research has confirmed that mental events are physical events at the same time—because every one of your thoughts activates a messenger molecule in your brain, where it is instantly, automatically transformed into biological information. It's not that a mental event of the thought causes the physical event of the molecule; rather, the mental event and the physical event *are exactly the same thing*. The thought is the molecule and the molecule is the thought. It isn't that one becomes the other or that one influences the other—the two are exactly the same event viewed from different perspectives.

So we should stop looking at the human body as a body and a mind, or as a mind inside a body, and view it instead as a *body/mind*. Furthermore, we should acknowledge the fact that the mind is not located only in the brain. Consciousness is the distinctive expression of the mind, and behavior that expresses consciousness is actually present throughout the body, in each and every cell.

Do you see how fundamentally these ideas can alter our perception of the experience of living? For all of your life, perhaps, you could look out the window and say, "Oh, that's the world." And to your old way of thinking, the world "out there" would be separate from the space "in here"—the space inside you, inside your skin.

You saw yourself as a skin-encapsulated ego. This was your personal body, and anything outside your skin was the world. But the fact is, this is a very artificial distinction. The world is my cosmic body and the space inside my skin is my personal body, and the two are *essentially the same*. They are part of the same continuum. It's artificial to divide one from the other just because my skin comes in between. Skin, of course, is made of the same fluctuations as everything around it.

So we're part of this continuum of nature—which is intelligent and self-referring—and this is the basis of Ayurveda. Ayurveda says: As is the atom so is the universe; as is the microcosm, so is the macrocosm; as is the human body, so is the cosmic body; as is the human mind, so is the cosmic mind.

Some people are uncomfortable with phrases like *cosmic mind* because of the spiritual connotations. But the cosmic mind is just a simpler way of saying a nonlocal field of information with self-referral feedback loops of a cybernetic nature. It's just two frames of reference expressing the same thing. Similarly, the rishis of India, who were the originators of the science of Ayurveda, didn't use the terminology of modern physics. They certainly understood the quantum mechanical body, but they expressed it differently, as a subtle body and a causal body.

But the basis of the rishis' thinking was the same as that of today's quantum physicists. Physical events are simply the expression of nonphysical events. These nonphysical events are particular bits of energy and information coming out of a field of energy and information. Just as we have a subtle body, we have subtle senses. Everyone has had the experience of closing their eyes and seeing the image of their mother, or a rose, as a subtle sense of vision. Where is that image? It's in that field of information.

You can prove this right now. Close your eyes and remember the taste of strawberry ice cream. The taste is *there*, certainly— but where is it exactly? It's in the subtle body. In the same way, you can close your eyes and hear music if you want to, or the feel of a woolen scarf around your neck. So for each of the five senses we have subtle senses that are also fluctuations of energy and information in the subtle body. And these senses—which are the subtle senses, the subtle body, the quantum mechanical body—give rise to the physical body. The physical body is nothing other than the expression of this subtle body, which is part of a universal field of information.

The dual properties of subtle body and causal body aren't unique to human beings or even to living things. The Earth also has its subtle body, as does the universe as a whole. The cycles of nature of our individual physiology and the cycles of nature of our cosmic physiology are part of a continuum; they match each other. The intelligence of nature is the same intelligence that operates inside us.

Ultimately, all of nature comes from this void. Inside us it is our own inner space, and outside us it is outer space. But this outer and inner space is not simply a void, it's the womb of creation, whence everything comes. And nature goes to the same place to create a thought, an idea, or a philosophy as it goes to create a liver, heart, or brain, or to create a galaxy, a rain forest, or a tree or a butterfly. Nature is intelligent. It behaves with certain rhythms and cycles of rest and activity. These repeating cycles occur in our body/mind as our own biological cycles. Scientists call them circadian rhythms, the twenty-four-hour cycle of day and night.

CIRCADIAN RHYTHMS

If, as we've suggested, the human body is like a river, constantly in the process of change, then it should come as no surprise that your body is not the same at seven o'clock in the morning as it is at seven in the evening, for example. This is true at the quantum level, but it's also something you experience directly through your perceptions. All of us have surges of energy at certain times and bouts of fatigue at other times. Your appetite is always in the process of change, and so are your cycles of rest and activity, sleep and wakefulness.

Science has long been aware of the cyclical character of nature at every level and certainly at the level of human experience. As the Earth goes around the sun, our bodies change with those cycles. So we may feel like we're falling in love in spring or getting depressed in winter, and that's because the biochemistry of the body changes as the Earth transforms itself in these cycles. Other cycles also influence us. The lunar month influences us through tidal rhythms because it's the same intelligence operating everywhere.

How does this influence the sleep patterns of any individual? In order to understand this, consider how far our contemporary way of life has taken us from the natural rhythms that governed human experience until surprisingly recently.

Once our activities, especially our daily labors, were measured by the rising and setting of the sun. A farmer worked in the fields until darkness fell, then he went home. And women's lives, by and large, were governed by the requirements of their husbands. Obviously, all that is very different now. We get up and go to bed by the clock, not by the sun. (This is an extremely significant development, of which you'll learn more in chapter 4.) Almost no one works in the fields anymore, having moved inside to offices of concrete, steel, and glass, where the windows don't open and hot or cold air is pumped in. When darkness falls, it's a simple matter to switch on the lights and keep working.

In short, our lives have gotten out of balance with nature's rhythm—and sleep is most definitely one of those rhythmic cycles. Living in harmony with natural rhythms allows a free passage of biological information and intelligence, while living in opposition to those rhythms fosters disorder at the molecular level and discomfort at the level of everyday experience.

Sleep is simply a naturally existing state of consciousness that should come in its own proper cycle day after day, year after year. It's the period of rest where rejuvenation and healing take place. Once you break free of the artifical imperatives of modern life and reestablish balance on the level of the quantum mechanical body, it's inevitable that sleep and all other physical functions will improve. Rather, not just better, but *perfect*. Because that perfection is inherent in nature. It can only become imperfection if in some way we interfere with fundamental truth.

In this book, therefore, you will not only learn how to get a better night's sleep, but by doing so you'll discover how to get back in touch with yourself, with your own perfect design. You will learn how to live in harmony with the cycles of nature, riding the waves of nature's rhythms. And it's not going to be difficult at all, because all you have to do is to get back in touch with the natural forces at work within you.

All sleep problems and many diseases occur because we are no longer synchronized with this self-referring part of nature's intelligence, which is one of effortless ease and bliss and happiness. Sleep is such a basic experience that improving it will automatically take you to a higher, more fulfilling experience of life.

A Practical Approach

to Sleep

Now, while always keeping in mind the larger perspective we explored in chapter 1, let's introduce some practical methods you can use for creating better sleep. All the techniques in this book are based on a single idea, which in my opinion is the single most important fact about this subject: *You cannot force yourself to sleep.*

You can't will sleep. You can't command sleep. You may have thousands of employees at your beck and call, you may be president or the queen, but you can't make yourself go to sleep in anything like the way you can make yourself climb a stairway or memorize the multiplication tables. It just won't work. The ancient Persian king Xerxes whipped the ocean when it refused to obey him. By trying to force it to do your bidding, are you trying to "whip" sleep?

Of course, with insomnia so prevalent, most of us have tried to force ourselves to sleep at one time or another. Now, in the daylight, there seems something comically absurd about the very idea. But it's not funny when you're tossing and turning night after night, *demanding* sleep from yourself, all to no avail.

Sleep is a natural process, and "trying" will have no positive effect. Trying will probably aggravate the insomnia, because the harder you try and the less successful you are, the more frustrating the whole enterprise becomes.

There's a very profound reason for this: Trying is not the way nature functions. The Earth doesn't *try* to go around the sun, nor does the seed *try* to sprout into a sapling. Nature functions with effortless ease, invariably taking the path of least resistance. This is the principle of least action and maximum efficiency, and it's the one to use when we want to fall asleep.

Therefore, the attitude you should adopt once you've gotten into bed is that which I call "not minding." The key to achieving this frame of mind is a total lack of self-consciousness. In other words, don't watch yourself, don't monitor yourself, don't become a commentator on your dilemma, and, above all, don't keep looking at the clock.

Instead, just rest comfortably, not minding, and use this attitude as a way of placing yourself in nature's hands. Simply lie in bed with your eyes closed, not minding whether you're awake or asleep. The mere act of remaining motionless with your eyes closed, even if you're feeling anxious or restless, actually provides the body with significant benefits.

SLEEP STATE MISPERCEPTIONS

People are notoriously inaccurate judges of their own sleep behavior. You may be getting considerably more sleep than you think you are, or a great deal less. For example, despite the fact that you can't force yourself to fall asleep, you may be able to trick yourself into it. You may already have done so many times without even knowing it.

Experiments have shown that individuals who have sleep problems often think that they have slept much less than they actually have, based on their EEG and polygraph measurements. This is called sleep-state misperception, or subjective insomnia. It's so common among people who complain of insomnia that sleep-disorder clinics report fully *half* of all people who can't sleep only *think* they can't. These delusions are present even regarding the details of a sleeper's misery. People who believe they were unable to close their eyes all night were actually asleep much of the time!

A study at the University of Chicago documents this phenomenon. Two self-described mild insomniacs were compared with a control group of thirty-two normal sleepers, matched for age, sex, and other characteristics.

After several nights in the sleep lab, the insomniacs reported that it took them an average of one hour to fall asleep. According to the lab instruments, however, they dozed off in only fifteen minutes. While the insomniacs did experience more wake-ups during the night than the control group, the disparity was nowhere near as great as they imagined: five and three-quarter hours of sleep compared with six and a half for the controls.

This peculiar phenomenon of subjective insomnia is one of the easiest sleep disorders to treat. And there's no doubt that it *is* a disorder, since the subjects do in fact feel sleep deprived and tired all day. In some experiments, they've even insisted that the instruments were wrong and that they never closed their eyes all night.

The solution to subjective insomnia is to turn the clock, so often the insomniac's worst enemy, into an ally. If you believe you lie awake night after night, see if you can prove it to yourself. Keep a notebook beside your bed, and glance at the clock occasionally—not at regular intervals but whenever the urge occurs—and write down the time. After recording several intervals ten or fifteen minutes apart, many people are startled to find that several hours have suddenly passed—and passed in *sleep*. This procedure should help eliminate the perception of sleep deprivation, and along with it the symptoms of fatigue the following day.

In light of the apparent determination of many insomniacs to believe the worst, it's interesting to note a phenomenon psychologists call *secondary gain*. This is the notion that when a person has suffered from a problem like sleeplessness, alcoholism, or another chronic condition for long periods of time, there may be benefits built into the condition that the subject has come to depend on, even though he or she may not be consciously aware of them. These secondary gains can make the problem more difficult to resolve. For example, you might find yourself saying that you would get more done around the house if you weren't so tired all the time from lack of sleep—but since you *are* so tired, the leaky faucet just isn't going to get fixed.

There are also people who, far from using their insomnia as an excuse, see it as a source of pride and strength. A young lawyer working in a major New York law firm found himself competing against people who rarely left the office for weeks on end, sleeping at their desks only three or four hours a night. "It was impossible to keep up with those people," the young lawyer said, "but their attitude was, 'How can I put my need for sleep ahead of the needs of the firm?' "

According to Dr. Peter Hauri, director of the Insomnia Program at the Mayo Clinic, some patients consider their inability to sleep a sign of concern for the world's problems: "How can anyone fall sweetly to sleep in a world as miserable as ours?"

There's a reverse side to these misperceptions of sleep time. Some people think they've slept quite well when in fact they may have slept very little.

Researchers have evolved an efficient system for identifying this phenomenon. A well-rested, healthy person requires between ten and fifteen minutes to fall asleep after getting into bed at night. But a sleep-deprived person loses consciousness almost immediately—although he or she is very unlikely to sleep through the night. Indeed, a sleep-deprived person doesn't have to be in bed to fall asleep right away. In research conducted by Dr. Thomas Roth, of Henry Ford Hospital in Detroit, one hundred young adults were asked to rate their level of daytime sleepiness and were then tested for sleep-deprived behavior. Thirty-four percent of those who said they weren't sleepy at all exhibited signs of severe sleep debt.

So, by lying quietly in bed, you may be getting more sleep, or less, than you think you are, but at least you'll be getting the significant rest that comes from just being still. Don't worry about whether you'll be able to perform well at work the next day. Studies show that, at least in the short term, people can carry out everyday tasks in normal ways even though they may not get enough sleep.

Go to bed at a regular time—we'll discuss this in more detail in chapter 4—and once in bed assume a comfortable position and don't worry about sleeping. Let your mind wander freely. Take the attitude that you will get as much rest as nature wants you to have at that moment, as much as you need, even if you're not actually sleeping. You are in nature's hands. Unplug your reading lamp; turn your clock to the wall; don't be concerned about the time. Just enjoy resting comfortably. Sleep will come naturally when it comes, and meanwhile you're gaining the benefit of valuable rest and rejuvenation of your whole system.

TOSSING AND TURNING

Often it is quite uncomfortable to be lying in bed unable to sleep. The mind may be racing, and there may even be physical discomfort throughout the body. In that case, just let it happen. Remember that the purpose of sleep is to dissolve fatigue and stress from the system. There is an old Ayurvedic saying: Sleep is the nurse of all living beings. Sometimes repair is overdue. Perhaps a great deal of stress has accumulated and now needs to be released during the night. This repair work, or release of stress, can increase mental and physiological activity, which may be experienced as physical discomfort, racing thoughts, or feelings of anxiety. If this is your experience, you should recognize these sensations of restlessness as a by-product of nature's repair work and not try to resist them or be worried about them. Instead, rest as comfortably as you can with your eyes closed, just not minding at all. Allow your mind to be easily aware of your body, and let the self-repair process go on.

You may find from time to time that you have a sensation at a particular point in your body. If this happens, your awareness should move easily to that sensation. Whenever there is turbulence in your mind, there is a corresponding turbulence in your body. For every mental event there is a physical event, and emotion is nothing but a thought attached to a sensation. When you shift your attention from thoughts to sensations, you dissipate the strength of the emotion, because thought and sensation are no longer chained together. You uncouple the two. Therefore, you can contribute to your attitude of not minding by just allowing your awareness to shift spontaneously to the sensations in your body—and then spontaneously to the thoughts and ideas that accompany those sensations.

After some time, the physical discomfort will abate and your awareness will move to some other thought or other part of your body. Just allow this to happen as spontaneously as possible. This simple procedure of allowing your awareness to shift from one sensation to another—just being aware of the sensations, the thoughts that come and go—is in itself a very powerful and profound anti-insomnia technique. Before you know it, your awareness will spontaneously have moved from thoughts, ideas, and sensations to a deeper, self-referral state of sleep.

DON'T GIVE UP AND DON'T GET UP

Remember that even if you are feeling quite restless, the best thing you can do is just rest easily in bed, eyes closed. Although the suggestion has been made that people experiencing sleep difficulties should read, watch TV, or get up out of bed and otherwise occupy themselves until they feel genuinely tired, I think this is a mistake. For one thing, it ignores the real benefits that the body derives just from resting quietly. Getting out of bed to read or do your taxes will interfere with the valuable process of rest and self-repair that was already taking place. Also, while getting up may provide temporary relief from the unpleasant experience of lying there awake, in the long run it is not the solution to the problem of not getting enough sleep. And, of course, it also ignores the phenomenon of subjective insomnia, which we've just discussed.

So "not minding" should be the attitude that you develop toward sleep. As you gain more knowledge and follow more Ayurvedic recommendations, you will find it easier to follow this first one.

MAKING A SLEEP CHART

Documenting your sleep patterns is an important early step in confronting your insomnia. It can be done with the aid of a simple chart, which can help you keep track of what is really happening with your sleep. The chart allows you to record the date, the time you turned out the light, the approximate times that you actually slept and awoke, and the times you actually got out of bed. You can also create a column for special comments or observations you may have about that day.

Filling out the chart each morning when you get up will not only help you document your progress but will help point up the relationship between certain activities or changes in your daily routine that may be influencing your sleep and hindering your progress. For example, during one particular week you may record that you had night classes and more stress at work, and then note the following week your sleep was more disturbed. On the other hand, you may find that as you follow the recommendations from this book you'll be able to track which recommendations had the most powerful effect on your particular sleep problem. You should continue to fill out the chart every morning until your sleep problem has been permanently solved.

THE FUNDAMENTAL SOLUTION TO INSOMNIA

Now you've got a technique to use when you go to bed: rest with closed eyes and let your awareness drift from sensation to sensation or thought to thought in a nonminding attitude. The more adept you become at using this technique, the better your sleep will be.

I want to emphasize once again, however, that the real solution for the sleep problems you encounter at night lies in what happens during the day. All these time periods are related, and to focus on one without considering the other can lead only to short-term solutions. Activity and rest go hand in hand, therefore we must pay attention to what happens during the day. If the period of activity is somehow imbalanced, that will be reflected in the period of rest.

The solution to all sleep problems lies in making the period of daily activity truly dynamic and satisfying. In other words, when you're awake, be *fully* awake. This is the fundamental answer to insomnia and the solution for many of the apparent problems of life as well. When you've learned to experience pure wakefulness, liveliness, and dynamism, good sleep will come naturally. Once you balance the activities of your life and

DAILY SLEEP LOG

Day   Date   Not asleep ••••••• Asleep ————

SLEEP PATTERN

8 9 10 11 12 1 2 3 4 5 6 7 8 9 10 11 12 1 2 3 4 5 6 7 8

•Daytime activities, how you felt:

_____

• Evening activities, how you felt:

_____

•Observations and conclusions:

Day   Date   Not asleep ••••••• Asleep ————

SLEEP PATTERN

8 9 10 11 12 1 2 3 4 5 6 7 8 9 10 11 12 1 2 3 4 5 6 7 8

•Daytime activities, how you felt:

_____

• Evening activities, how you felt:

_____

•Observations and conclusions:

Day   Date   Not asleep ••••••• Asleep ————

SLEEP PATTERN

8 9 10 11 12 1 2 3 4 5 6 7 8 9 10 11 12 1 2 3 4 5 6 7 8

•Daytime activities, how you felt:

_____

• Evening activities, how you felt:

_____

•Observations and conclusions:

experience the enjoyment that comes with that balance, your sleep will spontaneously become balanced.

In short, as you proceed through this book you'll find that by solving your problem of insomnia, you'll be solving a lot of other problems in your life at the same time.

SUMMARY

1. Pick a reasonable (early) time to get ready for bed, and establish a soothing routine beginning at the same time every night.

2. Once you've gotten into bed, rest comfortably with your eyes closed, "not minding." Let your mind be easily aware of your body. Remember: You're getting valuable rest even if you're not asleep.

3. If you're feeling restless or fidgety, or if your thoughts are racing, recognize that even these feelings represent the process of healing that's taking place.

4. If there's an unpleasant or painful sensation anywhere in your body, focus your mind on the sensation itself. By shifting your attention from thoughts to physical sensations, you uncouple the two and dissipate the strength of any anxiety.

5. Each morning, use your Daily Sleep Log to record what happened during the night.

3

DISCOVERING YOUR

AYURVEDIC BODY TYPE

In order to reawaken your body's intelligence effortlessly and to reestablish proper sleep, you need to understand how your body functions. Our source of knowledge for this book comes from Ayurveda, which in Sanskrit means "the science of life." Ayurveda is the oldest tradition of knowledge having to do with health, originating more than five thousand years ago. With the information about Ayurveda in this chapter, you'll be able to identify your particular body type in accord with ancient principles and learn some of the strengths and vulnerabilities that are associated with that body type.

The concept of psychophysiological body types is one of the most important ideas in Ayurveda. Through it, we can see how our bodies are unique expressions of nature's intelligence. We've all had the experience of reacting to specific situations and circumstances differently from other people. One person can hear a little bit of criticism from somebody and not mind at all; another person may react very violently and angrily; a third person may start worrying about his or her self-image.

When I drink a cup of coffee, nothing happens because I happen to have a strong Kapha constitution; other people may have only two sips and their nerves get jangled. In other words, each of us possesses psychological, biochemical, emotional, and intellectual individuality. We are unique expressions of nature's intelligence.

This individuality, even though it's unique, is manifested along certain patterns, in that we all have certain propensities or tendencies to express ourselves in certain ways. These psychophysiological tendencies or propensities are organized in Ayurveda as body types, or, in Sanskrit, "doshas." Specifically, there are three basic doshas that emerge as expressions of metabolic tendencies in both our physical bodies and our psychological makeup. The three doshas are known in Sanskrit as "Vata," "Pitta," and "Kapha." Vata controls all movement in the body, whether it's the movement of thought or the movement of bowels, the vibration of vocal cords or the gesticulations of hands, or even the dance of DNA as it replicates. Pitta controls metabolism and digestion, and Kapha controls structure. All the cells of the body contain these three basic, abstract principles—the principle of movement, the principle of metabolism, and the principle of structure.

Your body must have Vata, or motion, to breathe, to perform peristalsis, which allows food to pass through the digestive tract, to circulate blood, to keep the heart beating, and to send nerve impulses from one part of the brain to another. It depends on Pitta, or metabolism, to process food, to activate enzymes, to properly metabolize food, air, and water through the biochemical pathways, and to keep the intellect functioning. It has to have Kapha, or structure, to hold cells together and to form muscles, fat, bones, and sinew. Nature needs all three doshas to build and sustain a healthy body; the final expression of the harmonious and smooth interaction of all three doshas culminates in your basic character, which Ayurveda calls *prakriti*. This determines your body type, which is like a blueprint that outlines the innate tendencies built in to your system.

Each of us is constituted differently in terms of the doshas. If you are a Vata type, that means Vata characteristics are more prominent in you; likewise for Pitta and Kapha types. In other words, one specific dosha is predominant in your nature. By knowing your body type you can focus more precisely on your diet and on the kind of exercise and daily routine that you should have, which is very important when dealing with any health problem, whether it's overweight or diabetes or arthritis or insomnia.

Certain body types are prone to certain types of disorders. Kaphas, for example, are inclined to overweight or even obesity. The Vata types are prone to insomnia, restlessness, and anxiety. Of course this doesn't mean that if you're a Kapha type you can't have insomnia or that Pitta types can't gain weight. Those disorders can occur in anyone, but it's the Vata dosha that becomes unbalanced to cause insomnia, just as it's the Kapha dosha that ultimately gets aggravated to cause overweight.

Let's discuss the body types one by one, in order to give you some idea which body type or combination you are. Understanding this will help you relate your psychophysiological tendency to the insomnia that you've been experiencing—keeping in mind, of course, that insomnia is ultimately an aggravation or imbalance of the Vata dosha.

VATA

Vata types are usually light, with a thin build. They perform activities very quickly, and their hunger and digestion can be irregular. They are particularly prone to insomnia because their sleep is light and interrupted. By nature Vata types are enthusiastic, vivacious, and imaginative. They are excitable, their moods can change quickly, and when they go out of balance the same properties of enthusiasm and vivaciousness and imaginativeness can manifest as anxiety, worry, insomnia, restlessness, irritable bowels, menstrual cramps, or migraine headaches. All these can occur when the Vata dosha gets imbalanced.

Vata types are very quick to grasp new information, but they also tend to forget easily. They have, as I mentioned, a tendency to worry, a tendency to constipation, a tendency to overexert, and they tire easily.

The basic theme of the Vata type is changeability. Vatas are quite frequently unpredictable, and their behavior is much less regular than that of either Pittas or Kaphas. Their variability, whether it's in size, shape, mood, or action, is their trademark. For a Vata, mental and physical energy comes in bursts, without steadiness. So it's very Vata to be hungry at any time of the day or night; to love excitement and constant change; to go to sleep at different times every night; to skip meals; to have irregular habits in general; to digest food well one day and poorly the next; to have bursts of emotion that are short-lived and quickly forgotten; to walk quickly.

Vata is the dosha for movement. Vatas are usually lithe and lean. They tend to have light or restless sleep that lasts less than seven hours. Their appetites are irregular, and they often suffer from digestive problems. They don't gain weight easily. Regarding their general health, they're often subject to minor illnesses such as headaches, colds, and unexplained aches and pains. Yet a balanced Vata person is engagingly cheerful and energetic.

Temperamentally, Vatas seem to thrive on new things. They are better at starting things than at finishing them. When Vata is out of balance, it manifests as a frustrating, overall restlessness.

Perhaps the most important fact about Vata is that it points the way for the other doshas. Since it goes out of balance more easily than Pitta or Kapha, Vata is responsible for the early stages of almost all disease. There's also a fundamental connection between difficulties with sleep rhythms and unbalanced Vata dosha. Therefore, regardless of your body type, it's extremely important for everyone to keep Vata in balance.

PITTA

Pitta types are medium in build, with medium strength and endurance. For Pittas, hunger is sharp, as are thirst and digestion. They tend toward anger and irritability when under stress. Their skin is usually ruddy, fair, often freckled. Pitta types have an aversion to sun and hot weather. They're enterprising characters who enjoy challenges, they're good speakers, and they have strong intellects. They find it very difficult to skip meals. If their meal is even half an hour late they get ravenously hungry and can lose their temper.

The basic theme of the Pitta type is intensity. Anyone who has bright red hair and a florid face contains a good deal of Pitta, as does anyone who's extremely ambitious or sharp-witted or outspoken or bold or argumentative or jealous. The combative side of Pitta is a natural tendency, but it doesn't have to be expressed when the dosha is in balance. When in balance, Pittas are warm and ardent in their emotions.

Pitta regulates the body's metabolism. Pitta types have strong appetites and excellent digestion. They may put on weight if they overeat, but they also take it off easily. Temperamentally, Pittas are inclined toward anxiety and worry. They go out of balance less easily than do Vatas, but they can place such high demands on themselves that they become irritable and combative.

As regards sleep, Pitta types come closest of the three doshas to sleeping the "normal" eight hours, and their sleep is usually sound. If insomnia occurs, it usually means waking up in the middle of the night feeling overheated.

KAPHA

Kapha types have a solid, powerful build. They have great physical strength and endurance and steady energy. They are slow and graceful in action. They display the characteristics of tranquillity, they have relaxed personalities, and they don't lose their tempers easily. If you examine them, you find that their skin is cool and smooth, often thick and pale and quite oily. Kapha types are slow to grasp new information, but they have very good retention. They tend toward prolonged, heavy sleep, so Kapha types generally do not suffer from insomnia. Their digestion is slow and mild, they have an affectionate, tolerant, and forgiving attitude, and they tend to be possessive and complacent. Kapha types tend toward obesity and low levels of activity when they are imbalanced.

The basic theme of the Kapha type is that they are relaxed. Kapha dosha, the structural principle in the body, brings stability and steadiness. It provides reserves of physical strength and stamina that have been built into the sturdy, heavy frames of typical Kaphas. They are considered fortunate in Ayurveda because as a rule they enjoy sound health. Moreover, their personalities express a serene, happy, tranquil view of the world. It's very Kapha, for example, to mull things over for a long time before making a decision, to wake up slowly, to lie in bed a long time, to need a cup of coffee upon arising. Kaphas tend to be happy with the status quo and to preserve it by conciliating others, to respect other people's feelings, with which Kapha people feel genuine empathy, and to seek emotional comfort from eating. Kapha types have graceful movements, liquid eyes, and a gliding walk even when they are overweight.

As mentioned earlier, Kaphas are unlikely to suffer from insomnia, and their sleep is usually deep and sound. When Kaphas do have a sleeping disorder, it's usually oversleeping. Kaphas tend to wake up slowly, even groggily, and to start their day slowly. In addition, they hold on to things, whether it's food or fluid or fat or sleep or relationships, especially when they're under stress.

THE THREE DOSHAS

Their Basic Functions   Their Qualities

VATA

Governs bodily functions   Moving, quick, light, cold,
concerned with movement   rough, dry; leads the other doshas

PITTA

Governs bodily functions   Hot, sharp, light, acidic, slightly oily
concerned with heat and
metabolism

KAPHA

Governs bodily functions   Heavy, oily, slow, cold, steady
concerned with structure and   solid, dull
fluid balance

TEN CONSTITUTIONAL TYPES

ONE-DOSHA TYPES

| Vata | Pitta | Kapha |

TWO-DOSHA TYPES

| Vata-Pitta | Pitta-Kapha | Vata-Kapha |
| Pitta-Vata | Kapha-Pitta | Kapha-Vata |

THREE-DOSHA TYPE

Vata-Pitta-Kapha

You can probably see yourself in one of the descriptions below. Learn to respect your Ayurvedic identity, and, for our purposes here, learn to respect its sleep-related needs.

Characteristics of Vata Type

- Light, thin build
- Performs activity quickly
- Irregular hunger and digestion
- Light, interrupted sleep; tendency toward insomnia
- Enthusiasm, vivaciousness, imagination
- Excitability, changing moods
- Quick to grasp new information, also quick to forget
- Tendency to worry
- Tendency toward constipation
- Tires easily, tendency to overexert
- Mental and physical energy comes in bursts

It is very Vata to
- Be hungry at any time of the day or night
- Love excitement and constant change
- Go to sleep at different times every night, skip meals, and keep irregular habits in general
- Digest food well one day and poorly the next
- Display bursts of emotion that are short-lived and quickly forgotten
- Walk quickly

Characteristics of Pitta Type

- Medium build
- Medium strength and endurance
- Sharp hunger and thirst, strong digestion
- Tendency toward anger, irritability under stress
- Fair or ruddy skin, often freckled

- Aversion to sun, hot weather
- Enterprising character, likes challenges
- Sharp intellect
- Precise, articulate speech
- Cannot skip meals
- Blond, light brown, or red hair (or reddish undertones)

It is very Pitta to

- Feel ravenous if dinner is half an hour late
- Live by your watch and resent having your time wasted
- Wake up at night feeling hot and thirsty
- Take command of a situation or feel that you should
- Learn from experience that others find you too demanding, sarcastic, or critical at times
- Have a determined stride when you walk

Characteristics of Kapha Type

- Solid, powerful build; great physical strength and endurance
- Steady energy; slow and graceful in action
- Tranquil, relaxed personality; slow to anger
- Cool, smooth, thick, pale, and often oily skin
- Slow to grasp new information, but good retentive memory
- Heavy, prolonged sleep
- Tendency toward obesity
- Slow digestion, mild hunger
- Affectionate, tolerant, forgiving
- Tendency to be possessive, complacent

It is very Kapha to

- Mull things over for a long time before making a decision
- Wake up slowly, lie in bed a long time, and need coffee once you are up

- Be happy with the status quo and preserve it by conciliating others
- Respect other people's feelings (with which you feel genuine empathy)
- Seek emotional comfort from eating
- Have graceful movements, liquid eyes, and a gliding walk, even if overweight

At the end of this chapter you'll find an Ayurvedic body-type test. When you take this test you'll find out where you stand in this psychophysiological body typing. Balancing the three doshas produces perfect coordination in mind and body and therefore integration of physiological functioning. This is the goal we are shooting for. It will produce normal sleep naturally, as well as produce a healthy waking state. Sleep disturbances have their source in imbalance of one or more of the three doshas.

One thing that is important to know about your body type is that the dosha most dominant in any individual is most often the one that will go out of balance. This is especially true of the Vata dosha, because Vata is quick and mobile and has the inherent property of easily going out of balance. When you think of the symptoms of insomnia, you'll see immediately that the Vata dosha is the one that generally causes sleep problems. This is because Vata is active, light, quick, subtle, and changeable. Too much Vata easily causes sleep disturbances. When Vata is overly active the mind will become restless and have difficulty in settling down. But as you review the qualities of Kapha, you'll see that these are the qualities we normally associate with sound sleep. Heaviness, steadiness, softness, dullness, even sweetness (we speak of sweet dreams, for example). So aggravated Kapha is almost never the culprit in sleep disorders. Pitta can frequently be involved in sleep disorders, although much less often than Vata.

After filling out the body type questionnaire, you may find that Vata was part of your body type and that you are either a Vata or a Vata-Pitta type. Because it is actually imbalance that produces the symptom of insomnia, any type could theoretically have a Vata imbalance and therefore have insomnia. However, Vata types, or Vata-Pitta types, will most commonly have the symptom. So Vata is the dosha that we must pay special attention to. Vata types also tend to worry and may overreact to situations during the day.

It's interesting to note that sleep physiologists have defined different types of sleepers, and this knowledge correlates nicely with Ayurvedic knowledge of body types. One striking example is a type that sleep specialists describe as *hyperaroused*. Sleep specialists describe this type of person as being nervous and disorganized as well as tending toward fretting and worrying and dwelling on problems long after they're over. This observation of sleep experts clearly pinpoints some of the mental characteristics of the Vata type but leaves out important physiological characteristics that accompany this type.

A final important observation to make in this chapter is that individuals require different amounts of sleep in order to feel fresh and rested. For this reason, forget any preconceived notions of how many hours of sleep you need. It's true that Kapha types need more and Vata types need less, but what we want to achieve for everyone is a balanced, fresh state of mind and body at all times. Nature takes care of the number of hours of sleep that fits your particular body type. We know we've solved the problem of insomnia when we wake up in the morning ready to take on the challenges of the world with vitality and energy.

AYURVEDA BODY-TYPE QUESTIONNAIRE

The following quiz is divided into three sections. For the first 20 questions, which apply to Vata dosha, read each statement and mark, from 0 to 6, whether it applies to you.

    0 = Doesn't apply to me

    3 = Applies to me somewhat (or some of the time)

    6 = Applies to me mostly (or nearly all of the time)

At the end of the section, write down your total Vata score. For example, if you mark a 6 for the first question, a 3 for the second, and a 2 for the third, your total up to that point would be 6 + 3 + 2 = 11. Total the entire section in this way, and you arrive at your final Vata score. Proceed to the 20 questions for Pitta and those for Kapha.

When you are finished, you will have three separate scores. Comparing these will determine your body type.

For fairly objective physical traits, your choice will usually be obvious. For mental traits and behavior, which are more subjective, you should answer according to how you have felt and acted most of your life, or at least for the past few years.

SECTION 1: VATA

	Does not apply		Applies sometimes			Applies most times	
1. I perform activity very quickly.	0	1	2	3	4	5	6
2. I am not good at memorizing things and then remembering them later.	0	1	2	3	4	5	6
3. I am enthusiastic and vivacious by nature.	0	1	2	3	4	5	6
4. I have a thin physique—I don't gain weight very easily.	0	1	2	3	4	5	6
5. I have always learned new things very quickly.	0	1	2	3	4	5	6
6. My characteristic gait while walking is light and quick.	0	1	2	3	4	5	6
7. I tend to have difficulty making decisions.	0	1	2	3	4	5	6
8. I tend to develop gas and become constipated easily.	0	1	2	3	4	5	6
9. I tend to have cold hands and feet.	0	1	2	3	4	5	6

	Does not apply		Applies sometimes			Applies most times	
10. I become anxious or worried frequently.	0	1	2	3	4	5	6
11. I don't tolerate cold weather as well as most people.	0	1	2	3	4	5	6
12. I speak quickly and my friends think that I'm talkative.	0	1	2	3	4	5	6
13. My moods change easily and I am somewhat emotional by nature.	0	1	2	3	4	5	6
14. I often have difficulty falling asleep or having a sound night's sleep.	0	1	2	3	4	5	6
15. My skin tends to be very dry, especially in winter.	0	1	2	3	4	5	6
16. My mind is very active, sometimes restless, but also very imaginative.	0	1	2	3	4	5	6
17. My movements are quick and active; my energy tends to come in bursts.	0	1	2	3	4	5	6
18. I am easily excitable.	0	1	2	3	4	5	6
19. I tend to be irregular in my eating and sleeping habits.	0	1	2	3	4	5	6
20. I learn quickly, but I also forget quickly.	0	1	2	3	4	5	6

VATA SCORE

SECTION 2: PITTA

	Does not apply		Applies sometimes			Applies most times	
1. I consider myself to be very efficient.	0	1	2	3	4	5	6
2. In my activities, I tend to be extremely precise and orderly.	0	1	2	3	4	5	6
3. I am strong-minded and have a somewhat forceful manner.	0	1	2	3	4	5	6
4. I feel uncomfortable or become easily fatigued in hot weather—more so than other people.	0	1	2	3	4	5	6
5. I tend to perspire easily.	0	1	2	3	4	5	6

	Does not apply		Applies sometimes			Applies most times	
6. Even though I might not always show it, I become irritable or angry quite easily.	0	1	2	3	4	5	6
7. If I skip a meal or a meal is delayed, I become uncomfortable.	0	1	2	3	4	5	6
8. One or more of the following characteristics describes my hair: • early graying or balding • thin, fine, straight • blond, red, or sandy-colored	0	1	2	3	4	5	6
9. I have a strong appetite; if I want to, I can eat quite a large quantity.	0	1	2	3	4	5	6
10. Many people consider me stubborn.	0	1	2	3	4	5	6
11. I am very regular in my bowel habits—it would be more common for me to have loose stools than to be constipated.	0	1	2	3	4	5	6
12. I become impatient very easily.	0	1	2	3	4	5	6
13. I tend to be a perfectionist about details.	0	1	2	3	4	5	6
14. I get angry quite easily, but then I quickly forget about it.	0	1	2	3	4	5	6
15. I am very fond of cold foods, such as ice cream, and also ice-cold drinks.	0	1	2	3	4	5	6
16. I am more likely to feel that a room is too hot than too cold.	0	1	2	3	4	5	6
17. I don't tolerate foods that are very hot and spicy.	0	1	2	3	4	5	6
18. I am not as tolerant of disagreement as I should be.	0	1	2	3	4	5	6
19. I enjoy challenges, and when I want something I am very determined in my efforts to get it.	0	1	2	3	4	5	6
20. I tend to be quite critical of others and also of myself.	0	1	2	3	4	5	6

PITTA SCORE

SECTION 3: KAPHA

	Does not apply		Applies sometimes			Applies most times
1. My natural tendency is to do things in a slow and relaxed fashion.	0	1	2	3	4	5	6
2. I gain weight more easily than most people and lose it more slowly.	0	1	2	3	4	5	6
3. I have a placid and calm disposition— I'm not easily ruffled.	0	1	2	3	4	5	6
4. I can skip meals easily without any significant discomfort.	0	1	2	3	4	5	6
5. I have a tendency toward excess mucus or phlegm, chronic congestion asthma, or sinus problems.	0	1	2	3	4	5	6
6. I must get at least eight hours of sleep in order to be comfortable the next day.	0	1	2	3	4	5	6
7. I sleep very deeply.	0	1	2	3	4	5	6
8. I am calm by nature and not easily angered.	0	1	2	3	4	5	6
9. I don't learn as quickly as some people, but I have excellent retention and a long memory.	0	1	2	3	4	5	6
10. I have a tendency toward becoming plump—I store extra fat easily.	0	1	2	3	4	5	6
11. Weather that is cool and damp bothers me.	0	1	2	3	4	5	6
12. My hair is thick, dark, and wavy.	0	1	2	3	4	5	6
13. I have smooth, soft skin with a somewhat pale complexion.	0	1	2	3	4	5	6
14. I have a large, solid body build.	0	1	2	3	4	5	6
15. The following words describe me well: serene, sweet-natured, affectionate, and forgiving.	0	1	2	3	4	5	6
16. I have slow digestion, which makes me feel heavy after eating.	0	1	2	3	4	5	6
17. I have very good stamina and physical endurance, as well as a steady level of energy.	0	1	2	3	4	5	6
18. I generally walk with a slow, measured gait.	0	1	2	3	4	5	6

	Does not apply		Applies sometimes			Applies most times	
	0	1	2	3	4	5	6

19. I have a tendency toward oversleeping, and grogginess upon awakening, and am generally slow to get going in the morning.   0   1   2   3   4   5•   6

20. I am a slow eater and am slow and methodical in my actions.   0•   1   2   3   4   5   6

KAPHA SCORE

FINAL SCORE

VATA   **PITTA**   **KAPHA**

HOW TO DETERMINE YOUR BODY TYPE

Now that you have added up your scores, you can determine your body type. Although there are only three doshas, remember that Ayurveda combines them in ten ways to arrive at ten different body types.

• **If one score is much higher than the others, you are probably a single-dosha type.**
> **Single-Dosha Types**
> Vata
> Pitta
> Kapha

You are definitely a single-dosha type if your highest score is twice as high as the next highest dosha score (for instance, Vata—90, Pitta—45, Kapha—35). In single-dosha types, the characteristics of Vata, Pitta, or Kapha are very evident. Your next highest dosha may still show up in your natural tendencies, but it will be much less distinct.

• **If no single dosha dominates, you are a two-dosha type.**
> **Two-Dosha Types**
> Vata-Pitta or Pitta-Vata
> Pitta-Kapha or Kapha-Pitta
> Vata-Kapha or Kapha-Vata

If you are a two-dosha type, the traits of your two leading doshas will predominate. The higher one comes first in your body type, but both count.

Most people are two-dosha types. A two-dosha type might have a score like this: Vata—80, Pitta—90, Kapha—20. If this was your score, you would consider yourself to be a Pitta-Vata type.

• **If your three scores are nearly equal, you may be a three-dosha type.**
> **Three-Dosha Type**
> Vata-Pitta-Kapha

However, this type is considered rarest of all. Check your answers again, or have a friend go over your responses with you. Also, you can read over the descriptions of Vata, Pitta, and Kapha on pages 27–35 to see if one or two doshas are more prominent in your makeup.

4

Getting in Tune
with Nature's Rhythms

Everything that happens according to nature ought to be considered healthy," wrote Cicero, the Roman statesman. Our bodies follow natural cycles or rhythms—or at least they were intended to. In contemporary society, with the realities of working, traveling, and all the possibilities for distraction and entertainment that are regularly set before our eyes, it's difficult to realize that a vast, orderly universe exists all around us, operating according to an intricately structured, almost symphonic rhythm. We may try to ignore that rhythm, but it still asserts itself even through the static of everyday life.

Your own sleep/dream/wakeful cycle is, or should be, an expression of this pervasive natural harmony. It can be seen almost everywhere, if one takes the time to look. Earth rotates on its axis every twenty-four hours. It takes 365¼ days to revolve around the sun. The moon takes twenty-eight to twenty-nine days to revolve around Earth. Tidal rhythms express gravitational effects of the sun and the moon. All this is on a grand scale, of course, and modern science has only recently begun to recognize the full extent to which these cosmic rhythms have a counterpart within the physiology of every human being. For instance, there is evidence that the point in her monthly cycle at which a breast-cancer patient undergoes surgery is a tremendously important factor in determining the outcome of her treatment. There is also important evidence that illnesses such as clinical depression are dramatically influenced by seasonal changes and even by different times of day.

In order to enjoy perfect sleep it is essential to understand the extent to which the cadence of our internal experience is influenced by the larger rhythm surrounding us, just as a dancer will be drawn to move in time with the beat of an orchestra. In fact, it's not an exaggeration to say that the internal biological rhythm that each of us perceives as his or her own is actually an expression of the external beat of nature. In other words, these external and internal rhythms are just two expressions of the same carefully ordered natural cycles. These cycles are found throughout the plant and animal kingdoms and have even been observed in isolated cells and unicellular organisms.

For example, studies have shown that certain plants, sensitive to the cycle of day and night, can be placed in a dark room for days at a time and still continue to open and close their leaves according to the cycle of day and night, though they have no direct exposure to sunlight. This demonstrates just how deeply these basic cycles are ingrained in every aspect of nature.

In terms of these cycles' influence on our everyday lives, there's one particular well-documented phenomenon that deserves our close attention. Scientists call it *circadian rhythm*, the pattern of biological cycles that recurs at approximately twenty-four-hour intervals. Many of your body's vital signs are governed by circadian rhythm: Neurological and endocrine functions, for example, follow a twenty-four-hour cycle, as do temperature fluctuations, hormone and enzyme production, electrolyte excretion, and sleep/wakeful cycle.

The importance of circadian rhythm was first established more than thirty years ago during a series of experiments in the basement of a Munich hospital. A group of volunteers was placed in a windowless room, isolated from all external clues as to the time of day or the day of the week. They were allowed to establish and follow their own schedules for eating and sleeping. This study and later ones revealed that the human body operates on a cycle of approximately twenty-five hours.

This is very significant, because it suggests that if our internal pacemakers are not reset on a regular basis, they will begin leading us toward a schedule further and further from what the world considers regular hours. In other words, within two weeks we could be eating breakfast at midnight and getting into bed at dawn.

If we look beyond superficial explanations to explore genuinely fundamental causes, irregularities in the internal biological clock stand revealed as one of the most significant causes of insomnia. It's interesting to note that this loss of synchronization between the individual and his or her natural surroundings is a relatively recent phenomenon, at least in the degree to which we experience it today, and for this I blame two innovations that are fundamental to the benefits we enjoy in contemporary life, but which are definitely enemies of the natural sleep that our ancestors enjoyed.

These two innovations, which appeared in America at almost the same historical moment, are the electric light bulb and the notion of standardized time.

THE BEGINNING OF MODERN TIME

Time as we know it began only in the nineteenth century, after the Civil War. Until then, most regions determined their own time based on the position of the sun as they experienced it. Thus, "communities that were miles apart were also minutes apart." This could lead to problems of interpretation and correspondingly confusing results.

For example, somehow, because of the way the sun appears to move across the sky from east to west, Sacramento, California, was more than three hours earlier than New York City—almost three thousand miles away—but Sacramento was also about four minutes later than nearby San Francisco. Railroads, like towns, operated according to different versions of the time, depending on the location of their hub cities, and train stations displayed a selection of clocks, one for each of the various companies.

It was the railroads, in fact, that finally brought about the change to standardized time. But the transformation didn't come easily, for there was little public dissatisfaction with the multiple-time system. Today we completely accept the idea of one correct time that governs our lives: The time isn't a matter of individual opinion or interpretation, it is supposed to exist somewhere, perhaps in Greenwich, England, and we can hear it repeated on the telephone or the radio. If you were to argue seriously about the time, you would undoubtedly be considered quite odd.

Yet it was only after ten years of meetings among railroad executives and assorted meteorologists that, on November 18, 1883, Standard Time went into effect with the dropping of a huge ball from the top of a building in New York City—a tradition that still continues on New Year's Eve. Not everyone was glad to accept the new innovation. Certain states even refused to follow the new standard, but the *Indianapolis Daily Sentinel* expressed what eventually became the hard reality of the situation: "The sun is no longer to boss the job. People—55 million people—now eat, sleep, and work, as well as travel, by railroad time."

Am I opposed to a system of standardized time? No, and it's a little late for that anyway, by any reckoning. I want to live in the same world as everyone else. Later in this chapter you'll learn how even the alarm clock, that anxiety-producing enforcer of the one true time, can be enlisted in the cause of better sleep. Yet in terms of reorienting us away from the natural rhythms of nature toward a man-made, machine-controlled, deterministic experience of external reality, the introduction of Standard Time is hugely significant.

LET THERE BE ELECTRIC LIGHT

From the would-be sleeper's point of view, there's very little to be said in favor of the electric light bulb.

After Edison's development of the light bulb in 1879, darkness as it used to be known ceased to exist. The gas lighting that illuminated urban homes before that year, and the oil lamps that burned in rural areas, were effective to a certain degree, but they had disadvantages that made it easy for people to turn them off and go to bed. For instance, reading for long periods was difficult by gas or oil, and they were dirty compared with electricity. Also, compared with just flipping a switch, there was a certain amount of effort, sometimes even danger, involved in using gas or oil. (Rather than deal with them, the nineteenth-century poet Emily Dickinson preferred to compose many of her works in total darkness.) But with electricity there was almost nothing to it. By the turn of the century, you could stay up all night reading the standardized times of the train schedules.

The introduction of electric light in the home was another important factor in distancing us from the natural cycle of day and night. But, by comparison, the effect on our sleeping habits of electric lighting *outside* was much greater still. For one thing, electric lighting of the streets greatly increased the level of safety people could expect when they went out at night. And electricity ushered in modern forms of advertising, which provided all sorts of inducements for going out. Theaters, restaurants, and even amusement parks were fully illuminated, inside and out, within a few years of the invention of the electric light bulb. And at the Columbian Exposition in Chicago, in 1893, the wonder of electricity brightened literally miles of consumer goods in a vast department store created especially for the fair.

Throughout history, people had stayed home at night and, among other things, slept. They lived mostly in the country, and those who didn't were too frightened of the poorly lit streets to take any chances. But by the beginning of the twentieth century, people were moving to the cities, and also moving further and further from the natural rhythm of light and dark, of sleeping and waking. They were certainly going out more, but they were probably sleeping less, and definitely sleeping worse.

RESTORING HARMONY

Remember that in Ayurvedic terms, irregularity and change-ability are qualities of Vata. The increasing divergence between our daily routines and the natural rhythms of life have been crucial in producing the sense of instability that arises from Vata imbalances. Today, this imbalance may be considered an epidemic.

There are enticing aspects of an irregular lifestyle that appeal to many people, but if the quality of your sleep has become a concern, you must learn to bring your body's rhythm back into harmony with the natural cycles surrounding you. For above and beyond any man-made distractions, the rhythms of nature still exist and assert their force: The sun continues to rise and set, the tides ebb and flow, and these phenomena remain immensely powerful and influential, whether we recognize them or not.

The rest of this chapter is devoted to helping you reset your biological clock to its regular, orderly functioning in accord with all the cycles of nature. This is a key element in our approach to insomnia.

Scientists have observed many different influences on our physiology throughout the daily cycle. Your body temperature, your weight, your fluid balance, and the various thermostats throughout your body all undergo changes from minute to minute, from hour to hour. But Ayurveda says that there are master cycles in us governed by the quantum mechanical body and that each day we pass through these various cycles, which can be defined in terms of Vata, Pitta, and Kapha.

There are three cycles, each predominantly influenced by a different dosha, that take place from sunrise to sunset, and they repeat themselves from sunset to sunrise. The approximate times are as follows: From *6:00 to 10:00*, A.M. or P.M., an influence of Kapha is dominant in the environment. From *10:00 to 2:00*, A.M. or P.M., an influence of Pitta is more dominant. From *2:00 to 6:00*, A.M. or P.M., an influence of Vata is dominant.

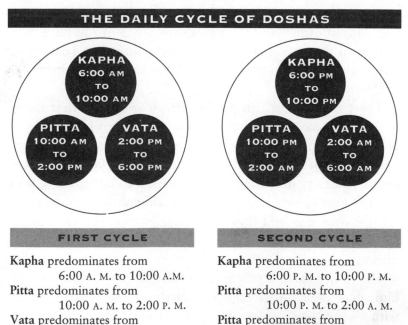

THE DAILY CYCLE OF DOSHAS

KAPHA
6:00 AM
TO
10:00 AM

PITTA
10:00 AM
TO
2:00 PM

VATA
2:00 PM
TO
6:00 PM

KAPHA
6:00 PM
TO
10:00 PM

PITTA
10:00 PM
TO
2:00 AM

VATA
2:00 AM
TO
6:00 AM

FIRST CYCLE

Kapha predominates from
6:00 A. M. to 10:00 A.M.
Pitta predominates from
10:00 A. M. to 2:00 P.M.
Vata predominates from
2:00 P. M. to 6:00 P.M.

SECOND CYCLE

Kapha predominates from
6:00 P. M. to 10:00 P. M.
Pitta predominates from
10:00 P. M. to 2:00 A. M.
Pitta predominates from
2:00 A. M. to 6:00 A. M.

One of the most basic aspects of living in tune with nature is to respect these master cycles that support our physical existence. We are not meant to fight against nature's waves; we are meant to ride with them, and our bodies experience a need to do that. It's only when we interfere with the process that we experience discomfort, whether from insomnia or anything else.

THE MOST IMPORTANT HOUR OF THE DAY

Simply by looking around, you can see the obvious influence of these natural cycles. We don't see birds awake at night except for owls, which have their own biological rhythm and their own purpose in nature's scheme. When we look around in the evening we see that nature is resting. As the sun sets, everything is quiet and nature settles down. We ourselves feel comfortable sitting back and relaxing in the evening. Of course, if you live in a large metropolitan area you may wonder where this silence in the atmosphere is as you look out on the dynamic activity of evening. However, this activity is not the influence that is present in nature itself, but is a part of our modern lifestyle, which brings us into conflict with nature itself. Observing nature, we find a settling, a heaviness and silence in the environment during this Kapha period of day. If we allow it, this will be reflected in our bodies also, which will feel heavy and naturally prepared for sleep. If we are in tune with this natural rhythm and heed this urge for rest as part of our daily routine, it's unlikely that insomnia will become a problem. But if we resist the desire for sleep, an entirely different pattern can begin to establish itself.

For this reason, *10:00 P.M.* is a pivotal moment in the entire twenty-four-hour cycle. This is the junction point between the Kapha and Pitta periods of evening. Ayurveda recommends going to bed at or before this junction time, because then the mind and body will be under the influence of the Kapha dosha. If you remember the qualities of Kapha—dull, heavy, slow, stable—

you will see that this influence in the environment is support-
ive of sleep.

What happens if you don't go to bed by 10:00 P.M., when the
influence of Pitta begins? By 10:30, this energizing influence has
become quite lively in the environment. Remember that Pitta is
an active dosha whose qualities are lightness, sharpness, and
heat, which imply activity. And this influence will bring out activity in you.

Most people find that if they stay up until 10:30 or later, they
can remain alert and mentally active until late into the night
with no difficulty. A certain kind of exhilaration even begins to
be felt. This is very clearly evident in children, who are so excited by the idea of "staying up late." It also accounts for the
fact that many creative people, whose art depends on the mental quickness and sharp juxtapositions of ideas, find it easiest
to work at night. The great French novelist Honoré de Balzac
was famous for sleeping all day, then waking up close to midnight to begin his work.

If you choose to stay up late, your sleep will be shallower and
less rejuvenating, and even this sleep will be more difficult to
achieve. Sleep researchers have established the fact that sleep
becomes lighter as the night progresses. This is absolutely con-
sistent with the Ayurvedic description of moving from Kapha
to Pitta to Vata—from heaviest to lightest—during the course
of the night.

THERE ARE NO NIGHT PEOPLE

An early bedtime is one of the most important points for bringing your system back into balance with nature, as it gives your
body the ideal opportunity for deep rest and normal sleep. Once
you're in bed, adopt the *nonminding* attitude discussed in
chapter 2. Above all, don't worry so much about falling asleep
that the worrying itself keeps you awake.

I had a patient who was seriously troubled by insomnia, and anxiety about it was only making the situation worse.

"I lie in bed every night until three-thirty in the morning," he told me. "After that I'm able to fall asleep occasionally, if I'm lucky. But never before three-thirty in the morning."

Fortunately, I was able to come up with a novel solution to his problem. "It seems like you're worrying too much and trying too hard," I suggested. "Just try to relax and do what comes easily to you. In other words, lie awake and don't allow yourself to go to sleep before three-thirty in the morning. Look at the clock every once in a while in order to keep track of things, but don't go to sleep before three-thirty."

"But that's what happens anyway," he protested.

"Well, nothing else has worked," I replied. "Just think of it as an experiment. You've been trying to do something that seems very difficult, which is going to sleep, so now give yourself the positive experience of doing something easy, which is staying awake."

This idea had immediate success. My friend was asleep long before 3:30 A.M. When he removed the necessity for going to sleep and placing it instead on staying awake, the tension that had been present every night was defused, and sleep happened all by itself.

If you're spending more time every night worrying about sleep than actually doing it, you might want to try the suggestion I offered to my patient. But I'm confident that for most people, an early bedtime and a nonminding attitude is the best approach. Of course, the very thought of this will make many people uncomfortable. Some may even react with a feeling of hopelessness or despair, as if you were asking the impossible. Others may say, perhaps even with some indignation, "I'm a night person, and I've always been one. I have more energy at night, and I have no desire at all to go to bed early."

Of course, Ayurveda teaches that this is a misperception, that there is really no such thing as a night person. There's only a

person who may be out of synch with his or her natural biological rhythms. If you have insomnia, this is certainly one of
the reasons for it. Over the years, many habits may have built
up that help to reinforce not going to bed early. These may include late-night reading, radio talk shows, and television.

But the truth is that you're paying a significant price for this
nighttime activity, not only in the short term but also because of
the diseases and imbalances that can arise as a result of deviat-
ing from your natural biological rhythms. After all, nature dic-
tates that up to one-third or more of our lifetime is invested in
sleep. We must demand the maximum return on that investment.

If you've become used to staying up past midnight, it's per-
fectly reasonable for you to feel wide-eyed and full of energy
and enthusiasm at that time. This is because long-established
habits of staying up late have influenced your biological mechanisms in such a way that you do in fact experience peak
energy and concentration at that time, even if it's achieved at
the cost of "sleepwalking" through the day. But if you'll go
along with my suggestion of early bedtime for a little while,
you'll realize that once you manage this change, your rhythms
will fall into synchrony with universal rhythms, and any temporary disorientation you experienced will have been well
worth the price.

You don't have to make this transition overnight, so to speak,
and it would be unwise to try, because you've been keeping
late hours for a long time. But once your internal clock has
been reset, I guarantee you'll feel an amazing surge of energy
in your daily experience—such buoyancy, such enthusiasm,
such liveliness, such wakefulness, such creativity. You'll enjoy
so much more in life by being fully awake. Today many people
are physically awake, but they're not really awake; they're
not fully aware. They don't have life-centered, present-moment
awareness.

The French philosopher Montaigne wrote, "When I dance,

I dance. When I eat, I eat." It sounds so simple, but are you really *there* when you're there, whether it's a place or a moment in time? So much in the contemporary world undermines our ability to be truly in the present, which is a crucial element of enjoying life.

Insomnia, which so often is filled with regrets about the past and worries about the future, is in a sense the exact opposite of living life with a present-moment focus. Despite the "high" you may experience from living like a night owl, it's no exaggeration to say that insomnia is something you *must* overcome before you can get the most out of every moment.

JET LAG WITHOUT LEAVING HOME

Many people suffer from what researchers call *Delayed Sleep Phase Syndrome*, which simply means that your internal biological clock has become mis-set over the years due to irregularities in your daily schedule, your diet, and other areas of your life.

As a result of this faulty internal clock, your system functions as if you were traveling from Los Angeles to New York on an airplane and were suddenly asked to go to bed at 10:00 P.M. New York time. Since your biological clock is set for three hours earlier, your body thinks it's 7:00 P.M. and finds it very difficult to go to sleep. People who make this trip often end up going to bed at about 1:00 A.M. because they feel as if it is 10:00 P.M. Which is, of course, the common phenomenon of jet lag.

Some people, however, develop a similar disorder of their internal clock while at home. We've already seen how the introduction of electric light helped foster this, but that was only the beginning. In ancient days, people's activities in their homes were very limited. Today, such activities are almost *un*limited, with so many new electronic devices coming along every year.

And, whatever their benefits in entertainment or the accessing of information, all of these novelties are helping to produce individuals whose natural biological rhythms are further and further out of sequence with the rhythms of nature, especially the rhythms of dark and light, than was true of any generation in the past.

With everything we've discussed stacked against it, preparing for a proper bedtime may at first seem a thoroughly foreign activity. Here, then, are five specific recommendations for evening and pre-bed activities:

1. *Supper should be light and should be eaten relatively early;* between 5:30 and 7:00 P.M. is best, as a heavy or late supper will take a longer time to digest. Digestion involves increased metabolic activity, which works against settling down for sleep.

2. *Take a short stroll after dinner,* about five to fifteen minutes, to promote relaxation and to aid digestion.

3. *Avoid exciting, dynamic, or focused activities in the evening.* Try to keep this a settled, relaxed time. Many people find that they get wound up during the evening, then have trouble unwinding and falling asleep. If you must attend to some focused activity or work at night, stop by 9:00 P.M. at the latest. Don't feel you've got to get everything done before you go to bed. If you have a good night's sleep, you'll have more energy, greater clarity, and greater success the next day.

4. *Avoid watching TV in the evening.* This may seem a tall order for many people, but it actually is very helpful for anyone who has a sleep disorder. If you must watch television at night, stop by 9:00 P.M. at the latest. TV, including programs that seem relaxing, is actually inherently exciting to the nervous system. It stimulates and even overstimulates sight, hearing, and overall mental function, and this aggravates Vata symptoms. Try substituting some light reading, listening to music, playing with children, having friends visit, or other relaxed activities.

5. *Begin to prepare for bedtime at least thirty minutes before you intend to get into bed.* Whatever routines you have before bed, such as brushing your teeth, as well as those you have added from this course, should be begun early enough to allow you to turn off the lights at your predetermined time. If you like to read before bed, do so in a room other than your bedroom. The bedroom should be associated with sleeping, not with mental activities such as reading or watching television.

These are some of the most important points in preparing for bed. But if, after reading them over, you still feel it's impossible even to consider getting into bed by 10:00 P.M., simply begin to *wake up earlier.*

Ideally, of course, you should move up both your rising time and your bedtime gradually, by a few minutes every day, for a total of about fifteen to thirty minutes each week. Regardless of how you do it, however, one of the most important things you can do toward making your body want to go to sleep at 10:00 P.M. is to get up earlier. Even if you find yourself missing your bedtime, maintain the schedule faithfully with regard to your rising time by using an alarm clock. Continue until you have established a rising time between 6:00 and 7:00 A.M. If you're diligent in this, the progressively earlier rising time will naturally lead to a progressively earlier bedtime, even though there may be some lag between the two.

This may seem a burden in the beginning, with the alarm clock and so on, but once you make a habit of waking at 6:00 or 7:00 A.M., your body will naturally want to go to sleep at 10:00 P.M. You won't be able to resist it. A regular rising time is essential to anyone who wants to improve sleep patterns, because it sets the entire day's activity off on a regular footing. It may take a few weeks on this schedule to achieve your goal, but gradually resetting your biological clock will lead you in the perfect direction for balancing Vata, and for making this change a permanent and beneficial one.

In general, there are two important points about the time you arise. First, you should wake at about the same time every day—preferably by 6:00 A.M. and certainly by 7:00 at the latest. Remember that Vata, which is irregular, is balanced by anything that is regular. Thus, regular arising is the most important thing you can do at the start of the day to balance the Vata dosha and improve your sleep patterns.

Second, you should set your time of arising so that it coincides with the end of the Vata period, at the junction point between the Vata and Kapha periods of morning. This means around sunrise, or about 6:00 A.M., when nature makes its transition from Vata to Kapha.

If you wake up prior to this transition, mind and body will still be under the influence of Vata qualities. Remember, these include alertness, lightness, activity, and quickness of mental and physical functioning. In addition, clinical studies have shown that rising early helps to alleviate depression. Awakening at this time prepares your mind and body for dynamic and effective functioning and clear mental activity during the day, which in turn sets the stage for sound sleep the following night.

If you sleep much beyond this time, you'll be sleeping into the Kapha period of morning. Awakening then will imbue the mind and body with the Kapha qualities of heaviness, dullness, slowness, and sluggishness. You have probably experienced feeling dull and sluggish during the day after getting up late in the morning. Much of the fatigue you may have attributed to lack of sleep can actually be the result of falling asleep late in the night and then waking up very late in the morning, disrupting your biological rhythms altogether.

WEEKENDS

To sum up: I suggest that you have a fixed time for arising and that you adhere to it, even if you must use an alarm clock, as part of your program of resetting your biological clock. This applies to weekends and holidays as well.

In fact, one of the biggest aggravators of sleep problems is changing one's wake-up pattern from workdays to weekends or holidays. That's why Sunday night is often a very likely time for insomnia. You may have slept late over the weekend, and now the prospect of work, with its attendant anxieties, has reappeared—and since you aren't tired due to sleeping late, you can't get your eyes to close.

Once you set the alarm for a fixed rising time, get up then no matter how much or how little sleep you feel you've had or how tired you feel. Even if you have enjoyed little or no sleep, continue to follow your normal daytime work schedule. Studies show that even tasks that involve fine motor skills are not generally affected by sleep loss unless it continues for an extended period. So even if you feel mildly uncomfortable for a few days or even a week after beginning to wake up early, this will be more than made up for by the comfort you'll derive from getting better sleep in the future.

When you get your daily rhythm back into line, you'll begin to wake up spontaneously at the appropriate time, and you'll be able to stop using the alarm clock. It's interesting to realize that the process of awakening has plateaus, just as going to sleep does. The natural process of waking up doesn't happen all at once. It certainly isn't anything like getting jarred out of bed by an alarm. Instead, you begin to move away from sleep in three or four stages, drifting back and forth between waking consciousness and very light sleep a few times before you finally open your eyes.

This half-asleep state is a dangerous area for Vata dosha. If you start to awaken before six in the morning, when it's still a Vata period, your thoughts might start racing and you'll snap into a fully awake condition. If this happens too quickly, you won't feel rested. You can feel tired for hours, as though you hadn't slept at all during the night.

The process of awakening depends on specific biochemicals that need to enter your system gradually and in the proper sequence. If you snap awake like an electric light, or if it takes you too long to wake up, so that you feel heavy and groggy, you can be sure that your internal rhythm has not yet been stabilized.

LUNCH

Before we leave the area of daily routines, there is one more pivotal time I want to discuss: the lunch hour. This is the time to have the main meal of your day, because noon is the exact middle of the Pitta daytime period of 10:00 A.M. to 2:00 P.M. As we've seen, within the body, Pitta is responsible for metabolizing food, for distributing energy, and for more efficient physiological functioning in general. Pitta corresponds to the influence of the sun in nature, and it plays these same roles in the internal nature of an individual. So when the sun is at its peak around noon, there will be maximum support from the environment for the digestive processes in the body.

This means that if you take your lunch at this time of day, you can digest a larger quantity of food and assimilate it properly. This helps give maximum energy and avoids the need to take a large meal at bedtime, which would be more difficult to digest and would therefore not only interfere with sleep but contribute to the accumulation of impurities in the body.

For all these reasons, try to have your main meal at lunchtime, and if you're in the habit of eating meat or other heavy foods, plan to make them part of lunch rather than dinner. Taken in the evening, these foods will sit in your stomach, and your body will strain to digest them when it should be settled and sleeping. Since work responsibilities can get in the way of having lunch on the job, making this the main meal of the day will definitely involve some extra planning. But with some creativity you can always find a way to accomplish this very important aspect of the daily routine.

You will definitely notice the benefits, not only in improved sleep but in increased energy, enhanced well-being, and better health in general.

The following are important points about the Ayurvedic daily routine and how it can help reset your biological clock so that sleep becomes that effortless and deeply restful experience that you remember so well from the past.

NAPPING

The ability to drift off into a restorative nap, even under trying conditions, is characteristic of some famous men of action. Churchill was known to nap every afternoon no matter what else was going on; John F. Kennedy was also a confirmed napper. In fact, during the height of the Cuban missile crisis in 1962, Kennedy refused to stay awake any longer after several days of working nonstop, and instead insisted on getting a full night's sleep. This was surely a very wise decision.

If you feel tired during the day, it's certainly healthier to take a nap than to drink a double espresso—indeed, the afternoon siesta is basic to daily routine in a large part of the world. If you like to take naps, however, there are several things to keep in mind.

First, be aware of the difference between *deciding* to take a nap and simply having sleep suddenly descend upon you whether you want it or not. If the latter situation occurs, particularly if it does so frequently, you may be suffering from one of the clinical sleep disorders discussed in this book. In Ayurveda, the notion of intention is a fundamental part of any action. If intention is not present, the benefits of napping (or anything else) are nullified.

Second, keep your naps under thirty minutes in length. If you sleep longer than that, you'll enter the delta phase of deep sleep, from which awakening is most difficult. You'll feel groggy and irritable and probably worse than before you fell asleep.

Finally, if you nap more than once a day, whether intentionally or not, you should have a medical evaluation. Such tiredness can be a symptom of conditions that are beyond the range of this book.

5

TECHNIQUES FOR SOOTHING

THE SENSES, AND FIVE

PATHWAYS TO RESTFUL SLEEP

Overstimulating the five senses is a major cause of insomnia. On the other hand, when treated properly, the senses can be avenues to restful sleep.

Hearing, touch, sight, taste, and smell are the pathways through which we gain knowledge of the world. But I believe our five senses do even more than that. We are the metabolic end products of our sensory experiences. To put it another way, we literally *metabolize* our environment through our senses. Everything that you experience through your senses—every sound, touch, sight, taste, and smell—becomes the very molecules of your body.

When your eyes see something, in less than one-hundredth of a second that sight causes a change in the biochemistry of not only your brain but other parts of your body. If you see a violent incident, for example, this will bring about a change in your brain chemistry, and simultaneously there will be a release of adrenaline and cortisol elsewhere in your body, and as a result of those hormones *other* hormones are also released—insulin, glucagon, growth hormone—and many, many other changes will occur as well.

Remember, everything that you touch, taste, smell, see, or hear is metabolized. We human beings don't metabolize only food; we metabolize our sensory experiences and they become the molecules of our bodies. There's a Vedic expression that says, "If you want to know what your experiences were like in the past, just examine your body now. And if you want to know what your body will look like in the future, examine your experiences now."

I believe that is absolutely accurate from a biological viewpoint, because, as discussed, you are the metabolic end product of your sensory experiences. Moreover, the world that you perceive through your senses is in a fundamental way a product of you. That's because in addition to being receiving mechanisms for external stimuli, the five senses are at the same time five different projections of your consciousness, your inner awareness, and your intelligence.

These are the ways in which the self reaches out to the world around it. We like to think that the world around us is exactly as we see it or as we hear it. But that's not really true, because ultimately we and our surrounding environment are all composed of the same energy fields, the same information fields, the same quantum soup that is a radically ambiguous and ceaselessly flowing amalgam of energy and information.

In the very act of seeing, hearing, smelling, tasting, or touching, we freeze that swirling mixture into the recognizable objects of our perception. In a sense, we're each like King Midas, who could never experience the texture of a rose or the soft caress of a kiss because as soon as he touched it, it turned into gold. It's as if, behind your back, there's a constantly flowing quantum soup, and the moment you turn and look, it's transformed into ordinary material reality through the projection of your consciousness.

The five senses are expressions of streams of intelligence that flow from the ocean of infinite intelligence, the reservoir of cosmic knowledge, to become the objects of the world. The five senses are projections of ourselves; then we metabolize these projections and convert ourself into material bodies.

How this happens is really quite amazing, and the body's ability to metabolize sensory experience has many implications for the healing process. But for our purposes here, it should be obvious that imperfect use of your senses will create an imbalance in your physiology. Specifically, overstimulating some or all of the five senses leads to an agitated state of consciousness that cannot settle down appropriately at bedtime. And this can lead to all kinds of sleep disturbances.

The racing thoughts and restlessness of mind that frequently keep people from falling asleep originate in overstimulation of the senses. Because Vata is so closely related to all mental activity, overstimulation or hyperarousal of the senses commonly influences Vata and results in insomnia. The fast pace of modern life, as well as the many technological developments I referred to earlier, have made hyperarousal of the senses almost epidemic. In fact, it has become fashionable to overstimulate and strain our senses. If you have any doubt about this, just look in the newspaper's listing of the most popular movies playing in your area. In movies, the more graphic and more violent the scenes are, the more popular they become. In music, the more loud and jarring, the more popular that music. Sensory hyperarousal is one reason why Vata disorders such as anxiety syndromes and insomnia have become so widespread.

In the course of the research that's been done on sleep disorders, *hyperarousal insomnia* has emerged as a specific category of problem. The brain waves of people affected by hyperarousal insomnia, as measured by EEG, show significantly less alpha rhythm than those of the average person. Since the presence of alpha rhythm is associated with a wakeful but calm state of mind, in which the subject is alert but not easily agitated, it follows that hyperaroused individuals are driven thinkers and worriers. More specifically, they seem to have difficulty preventing the stimulation they encounter in one setting from having an impact on every other area of their lives. If a hyperaroused person has an argument with his or her spouse before leaving for work, job performance will be affected. And, of course, if he or she has a bad day on the job, there may be another domestic dispute in the evening.

There are questionnaires to help identify hyperaroused individuals, but if you are such a person, you probably know it already. Key characteristics are overreacting to minor disturbances, such as traffic jams or long lines at the supermarket, and an inability to put these experiences out of your thoughts, to drop them, once they're over. And, unfortunately, another defining element of the hyperaroused personality is frequent reliance on tranquilizers or sleeping pills in order to deal with the symptoms.

Drugs do not provide a real solution to the problem of insomnia. In fact, sleep-inducing medications are so ineffective in any real sense that it's difficult to understand why there continues to be such an overwhelming demand for them. In one research study, the sleep of drugged subjects who had been diagnosed as insomniacs was compared with the sleep of a control group of untranquilized problem sleepers. It was found that the pill takers awoke twice as often as the control group during the night. Even when the drugs did put them to sleep, EEGs showed that they experienced no deep sleep at all and less REM sleep than the drug-free group, who managed an average of at least forty-five minutes of deep sleep before waking up again. And although night-sleep deprivation does not normally result in measurably impaired performance the following day, this is not the case with individuals who take drugs. Frequently, sleeping pills have an impact on thinking ability and muscular coordination for days after they were taken.

In short, most such drugs are habit-forming and have potentially serious side effects; the sleep they produce is artificial or abnormal, and scientific research has documented that sleeping pills and tranquilizers do not have a genuinely beneficial effect in terms of correcting a sleep disorder. At best, they provide the individual with a sense that something is being done about his or her insomnia, but this artificial and unrealistic reassurance only masks the underlying problem, which is almost always a Vata imbalance. If you are currently taking drugs for a sleep problem, I recommend that you gradually discontinue them under your doctor's care as you implement the approaches offered in this book. It will probably be best not to undertake this withdrawal all at once. Allowing yourself four to six weeks for gradual discontinuation of sleeping pills would be a very reasonable approach.

THE FIVE SENSES

Ayurveda recommends certain measures and specific techniques to help promote balance through each of our five senses. Since sleep difficulties originate in unbalanced Vata, following these measures can benefit your sleep as well as other areas of your life. Following these recommendations is valuable overall but is especially important in the hours just before bedtime. I've arranged the recommendations according to each of the senses.

Hearing

According to Ayurveda, the human body is a manifestation of sound. More specifically, our bodies are expressions of primordial sound, or ancient natural sounds expressing themselves in rhythms and synchronicities and frequencies of vibration.

These frequencies of vibration become the energy fields that ultimately become the matter of our bodies. For the ancient sages of Ayurveda, these vibrations were literally the bond that held the universe together: an invisible force, but infinitely strong, like the power that keeps the electrons and protons of an atom in orbit around the nucleus.

The rhythms that are inherent in our bodies are in fact universal rhythms. Our biological rhythms are in fact part of the symphonic orchestra in which we participate. We are an instrument in the music of nature, and therefore our organs—the liver, the kidneys, the heart—each of them has its own music. When we develop instruments that will amplify the vibrations produced by each of our bodily organs, it will be seen that the body as a whole is a virtual symphony.

We each have a unique song to play in the music of the universe. When disease is present, there is a distortion in that song, and Ayurveda uses sound to correct the distortion. Therefore, hearing plays a very important role in rebalancing our biological rhythms. You should try, first of all, to avoid sounds that are overly stimulating or dissonant or otherwise unpleasant. This would include music that has a jarring effect. Research has shown that plants grow better when exposed to beautiful music and don't grow as well when exposed to loud or jarring music.

Music therapy is a specific branch of Ayurveda called *Gandharva-veda*. Gandharva-veda uses melodic sequences of sound to promote balance in the individual mind and body, as well as in the surrounding environment, which is our cosmic body. Gandharva-veda helps in the entrainment of individual biological rhythms to the cycles of nature. At the end of this book you'll find source information for acquiring a Gandharva-veda sample tape to benefit your sleep. This will help to entrain your rhythms into nature's rhythms and help facilitate the progression from waking state to drowsiness to deep sleep. If you are particularly restless in bed and completely unable to sleep, for example, you could listen to Gandharva-veda even in the middle of the night, keeping the music very soft for maximum benefit.

I've had patients who were able to fall asleep without any difficulty, but then found themselves waking up quite suddenly in the middle of the night, almost in a state of panic, and yet without the memory of a nightmare or anything of that sort to explain it. For no apparent reason, their hearts were pounding, their mouths were dry, and they had such a sensation of fear that it was difficult for them to fall back asleep for the rest of the night.

There are two procedures that can immediately benefit this particular kind of sleep disorder. The first is a technique I brought up earlier: Try to lie quietly, feeling the physical sensations that accompany the situation—trying to uncouple the feelings of fear and panic from the actual feelings of your heart pounding and your breath becoming short. The second procedure I recommend is listening to Gandharva-veda music. Once the initial sensation of panic has begun to subside, listen to the music with the nonminding attitude that's effective for bringing on sleep. Just create in yourself a simple awareness of the sounds, and when you feel your attention drifting elsewhere, gently bring it back to listening. This will pacify the Vata disturbance that is the basic cause of the problem.

Touch

Your skin is one of the largest pharmacies that you could possibly have access to. Next to the gastrointestinal tract, skin is the organ richest in healing substances, including immunomodulators, drugs like tumonecrosis factor, which is an anticancer drug, antidepressant drugs such as imipramine, and vasoactive intestinal polypeptide, which opens up blood vessels. So it is becoming clear to researchers that the skin is a major source of healing chemicals.

Most significant, we can put the resources of this pharmacy to use immediately because it's directly accessible to us through the experience of touch. Touch is a very important sensory element and is directly related to the Vata dosha. After all, Vata governs the activity of the nervous system, and the skin surface contains thousands of cutaneous nerves that allow easy access to this dosha. So every person needs a minimal daily dose of touch.

It's interesting that every neuropeptide, every neurochemical known to occur in the nervous system, is also found in the skin. In fact, the skin and the nervous system are very intimately connected. A single part of the developing fetus, known as the neuroectoderm, gives rise to both. As a result, you can alleviate a lot of anxiety and restlessness, which we usually think of as being solely confined to the nervous system, through the skin, because the two elements of your body are so intimately connected—*inseparably* connected, in fact, not only in terms of the nerves that go from the skin to the brain but even by the neurochemicals that make up the skin and the nervous system.

For this reason, Ayurveda recommends certain types of massage that help reestablish a balance of Vata through balancing the entire nervous system. A sesame oil massage to the entire body, called *abhyanga,* should be done on a daily basis. The warm, soothing quality of the sesame oil is especially good for balancing the cold, light, and dry qualities inherent to the Vata dosha. In general, Ayurveda recommends the oil massage in the morning before you bathe. In the case of severe insomnia, however, you should try switching the oil massage to the evening before bedtime and follow it with a warm bath. You may find this an excellent evening routine as part of preparing for a deep, good sleep.

An alternative to a total body massage before bed is to simply massage the bottoms of your feet with oil. If Pitta is your major dosha (see your results to the Body-Type Questionnaire in chapter 3), use coconut oil for the foot massage; otherwise sesame oil is best. The feet are said to contain many vital points that relate to balancing the nervous system. Massaging the feet with warm oil before bed balances these points and helps to promote sound sleep. You can sponge the oil off with a cool cloth after a few minutes. This will have a soothing effect, although not as profound as that of the total body massage.

There are also vital points called *marmas* all over the body. Two major marmas that relate to sleep are located in the center of the forehead and on the lower abdomen just below the navel, about three-quarters of the distance from the umbilicus to the pubic bone. Before bed, gently massage each of these areas with a small amount of sesame oil, or coconut oil for Pitta types, using very light, circular, clockwise motions. This should take only about a minute.

A final point about touch concerns the sensitivity of the skin to the surrounding environment. Try to avoid excessively dry or humid environments that produce discomfort. Your bedroom should be well ventilated, and the temperature should be on the cool side, about 68 degrees Fahrenheit, or cooler according to your level of comfort. Overly warm temperatures are known to disturb sleep. If you use an air conditioner, be sure that the cold air does not blow directly on your head, for this would increase Vata. Many people find that natural fibers are best for bedclothes and sheets.

Sight

Visual stimuli are potent exciters of the nervous system. As I previously mentioned, try to avoid television late in the evening, and specifically avoid shows and films that are particularly violent or graphic. Every influence in your life that has a hyperarousing effect will in a cumulative way influence your sleep. It's not necessary to become a recluse from the wide world of consumer electronics, but in the evening make an effort to limit yourself to productions that you can actually enjoy and that make you feel more relaxed and calm when you watch them.

The bedroom itself, of course, should be as visually pleasant as possible. Preferably, the window should look out on a scene of natural beauty. If this isn't possible in your location, studies have shown that just the sight of an aquarium with a few tropical fish swimming in it, or the presence of a beautiful painting, can have a much more soothing effect than looking out at a parking lot or a street full of traffic. This same effect has been documented by hospital patients recovering from surgery. Those whose rooms had a view of a lawn or trees healed much faster and were discharged earlier than were patients whose windows viewed the hospital parking lot or the street. So try to create an environment that is natural, wholesome, life-supporting, and pleasing to the eyes. Keep your bedroom clean, and be sure to make your bed each day, so that the last impression before retiring is one of harmony and orderliness. A color scheme that is warm and soothing is best for restful sleep.

If your body type is Pitta, these recommendations should be followed carefully, since the Pitta dosha is particularly sensitive to visual stimuli.

Taste

Taste is another avenue along which your body accesses the information field of the universe. In effect, the sense of taste acquires information from the environment, matches this information with the information fields in your own body, and thereby creates balance.

Your taste buds are exquisitely sensitive receptors that reveal the overall body's amazing sensitivity and profound intelligence. For example, if you make a dilution of sugar and water, your body can perceive it in a dose of 1 part in 200. Salt can be perceived in a dilution of 1 part in 400; sour taste in a solution of 1 part in 130,000; and bitter in a solution of 1 part in 2 million! This exquisite discernment of taste has been developed by nature to allow food to speak to our doshas, enabling us to perceive directly on the level of taste what nature is trying to tell us about our needs. In the next chapter, we'll consider the subject of diet in more detail, but it should be mentioned here that certain foods are identified by Ayurveda as having an inherently agitating effect, and they should be avoided by people who have insomnia. These include stimulants such as caffeine and nicotine and depressants such as alcohol. It would be best to avoid them as much as you can.

Warm milk has been shown to benefit sleep when taken just before bedtime, and Ayurveda recommends the addition of certain herbs to the milk to increase its sleep-enhancing effect.

Smell

I've chosen to consider this sense last because, more than any other sensory experience, smell influences our behavior, our memories, and many autonomic nervous system functions, which are below the level of conscious awareness. This is because the receptors in the nose, known as the *olfactory bulbs*, are direct extensions of a part of the brain known as the *hypothalamus*. The hypothalamus, which is also known as the brain's brain, is responsible for many functions in our bodies, particularly those that we consider autonomic: heartbeat, blood pressure, thirst, appetite, and, of course, the cycles of sleeping and waking. The hypothalamus is also responsible for generating chemicals that influence memory and emotion.

So right here in this small part of the brain, the hypothalamus, which extends into the nose at the olfactory bulbs, is the whole machinery that regulates memory, behavior, autonomic function, and the sleep/wake cycle. We have access to this part of the brain directly through the sense of smell.

For example, there are hormones called *pheromones* that influence sensations of pain and pleasure, and they are transmitted as odors in the environment. Our emotions influence the concentration of these hormones in our bodies, and we release them into our environment as a result of the emotional state we are experiencing. If you're excited or afraid, you release pheromones of fear or excitement into the air, and people nearby sense and respond to that on some level.

So when we speak of a room having a tense atmosphere, or of a home having an atmosphere of affection, this is not just a metaphor. It may be quite literally true, and you've become aware of that through your sense of smell.

Since emotional states can be so directly influenced through the sense of smell, certain aromas are useful for balancing and pacifying the doshas. Therefore, aroma therapy is an important technique for bringing about ideal sleep. Try a mixture of warm, sweet, and sour aromas that are Vata pacifying, which include basil, orange, rose, geranium, clove, and some other spices. In Western herbalist traditions, oil of lavender is considered especially effective for sleep. A drop or two rubbed on the forehead is the recommended application.

INDIVIDUAL DIFFERENCES

In this chapter we've seen that by metabolizing our sensory experience in a wholesome manner, and by restoring the memory of wholeness in the quantum mechanical body, we can make our sleep much more restful, much more blissful, much more beneficial to health. Waking activity will in turn be more dynamic and fulfilling.

Experience tells us that individuals differ in their receptivity to the various types of sensory input. For example, some people are most influenced by sound and would therefore be more receptive to techniques using the sense of hearing, such as music therapy. People more oriented toward the sense of touch will be more receptive to such techniques as the Ayurvedic oil massage, or marma therapy, the traditional Ayurvedic approach that enlivens vital points on the skin's surface. As you incorporate the recommendations from this chapter into your daily routine, fill out the Bedtime Checklist that follows in order to see which sensory techniques have the greatest benefit for you. Then you may want to deemphasize the techniques that seem to be least effective while incorporating the others into your routine.

How to Do Ayurvedic Oil Massage

1. Start with cold-pressed sesame oil, available from your health food store. Ideally, the oil should be "cured" before using. (Instructions for curing are given below.) The oil should be warmed each day before you use it. One easy way to do this is to keep the oil in a small plastic bottle with a flip-top lid. Warm the oil by placing the bottle in a sink filled with hot water for a few minutes.

2. Use the open part of your hand, rather than your fingertips, to massage your entire body. In general, use circular motions over rounded areas (joints, head) and straight strokes over straight areas (neck, long bones). Apply moderate pressure over most of your body and light pressure over your abdomen and heart.

3. Start with your head. Pour a small amount of oil on your hands and vigorously massage it into your scalp. Using the flat part of your hands, make circular strokes over your head. Spend more time massaging your head than other parts of your body.

4. Move to your face and outer ears, remembering to apply a small amount of oil as you move from one part of your body to the next. Massage this area more gently.

5. Massage the front and back of your neck and the upper part of your spine. At this point you may want to cover the rest of your body with a thin layer of oil to give it maximum time to soak in.

6. Vigorously massage your arms, using a circular motion on your shoulders and elbows and long, back-and-forth strokes on your upper arms and forearms.

7. Now massage your chest and stomach. Use a very gentle, circular motion over your heart and abdomen. You can start on the lower right part of your abdomen and move clockwise toward the lower left part to gently massage your intestines.

8. Massage your back and spine. Do not worry if you have trouble reaching parts of your back.

9. Massage your legs vigorously, using circular motions over your hips, knees, and ankles. Use long, straight strokes over your thighs and calves.

10. Finally, massage the bottoms of your feet. As with your head, this important area of your body deserves more time. Use the palm of your hand to massage your soles vigorously.

11. Follow your oil massage with a warm bath or shower.

How to Prepare Sesame Oil for Ayurvedic Oil Massage

Ayurveda recommends using unprocessed, cold-pressed sesame oil, which is available at health food stores. Before using the sesame oil, cure the oil by following these simple steps. Curing increases the oil's ability to penetrate the skin.

1. Heat the oil to about the boiling temperature of water (212° F). To know when the oil is hot enough, simply add a single drop of water to the oil in the beginning. When

the water crackles or boils on top of the oil, remove the oil from the heat. Or just observe the oil as it heats. When it begins to move and circulate in the pan, remove it from the burner.

2. If you like, you can cure up to one quart of oil at a time. This should be enough for at least two weeks.

3. Because all oils are flammable, be sure to observe proper safety precautions. Use **low** rather than high heat, never leave the room while the oil is heating, and remove the oil promptly once the proper temperature is reached. Be sure to store the oil in a safe place when cooling, out of the reach of children.

Restful Recommendations

- Try to avoid sounds that are overly stimulating, dissonant, or otherwise unpleasant.
- Massage the bottoms of your feet with warm sesame oil before bed. Sponge off the oil with a cool cloth after a few minutes. If Pitta is your major dosha (according to the Body-Type Questionnaire you took on pages 36–41), use coconut oil instead.
- Before bed, gently massage the two major vital points that relate to sleep (in the center of your forehead and the lower part of your abdomen). Use sesame oil (or coconut oil if you are a Pitta).
- Avoid excessively dry or humid environments. Keep your bedroom well ventilated and on the cool side. Do not sleep with cold air blowing directly on your head, as that will disturb the Vata dosha.
- Do a sesame oil massage (abhyanga) each morning before your bath or shower. If your insomnia is severe, try doing the oil massage before bedtime and follow it with a warm bath.
- Avoid watching television at night, especially after 8:30

to 9:00 P.M. Avoid violent films in general, as these disturb the Vata dosha.

- Keep your bedroom clean and neat. Use colors that are
warm, soothing, and restful.
- Avoid stimulants such as caffeine, nicotine, and alcohol.
- Drink a cup of warm milk before bed. To make milk more
digestible, Ayurveda suggests that you boil it before drinking. Also, it's better not to mix milk with sour or salty food.
So if you eat a meal that includes these tastes, wait about
half an hour before drinking milk.
- Continue using your **Daily Sleep Log** and the following
Bedtime Checklist to record your sleeping patterns and
nighttime activities. The simple act of recording your habits
will help you remember to implement the recommendations from this book.

- **Cardamom-Nutmeg Milk.** Pour one cup of milk into a
saucepan and bring it to a boil. After a moment, remove it
from the heat. Add two pinches of ground cardamom and
two pinches of ground nutmeg. Sweeten to taste with sugar.
It's best to use unrefined sugar (such as Sucanat), available
at health food stores.
- **Cardamom-Saffron Milk.** Use the same recipe as above, except add two to three threads of saffron instead of nutmeg.
- **NOTE:** You can add two pinches of grated or finely
chopped fresh ginger to the milk before you boil it. Fresh
ginger makes the milk more digestible. (Do not use pow-
dered ginger, however, as it is too hot and stimulating to
take before bed.)

BEDTIME CHECKLIST

Each morning, check off the recommendations you followed the night before to prepare your mind and body for sleep.

	Mon.	Tues.	Wed.	Thur.	Fri.	Sat.	Sun.
EVENING ACTIVITIES							
Ate an early, light supper							
Took a short walk after dinner							
Avoided focused work after dinner							
Avoided watching TV after dinner							
Enjoyed light, relaxing activities							
BEFORE GETTING INTO BED							
Allowed $1/2$ hour to prepare for bed							
Massaged feet (or full body massage)							
Massaged the vital points (forehead and abdomen)							
Drank a cup of warm milk							
Prepared aroma therapy							
Set alarm for 6–7 A.M. or earlier							
AFTER GETTING INTO BED							
Was in bed before 10 P.M. (if later, record time)							
Listened to Gandharva-veda music							
Adopted a "non-minding" attitude							
Woke up before 6–7 A.M. (if later, record time)							

BALANCING THE

PHYSIOLOGY

Insomnia can't be cured without treating the underlying imbalance that causes it. In this chapter you'll learn how to restore balance to your mind/body system through meditation, diet, exercise, and herbal food supplements.

All this will not only improve your sleep but foster success in every area of your life. Because insomnia, after all, is more than just a sleep disturbance. It is an expression of an overall imbalance in the physiology. According to Ayurveda, sleep is one of the pillars of health—so when sleep is disturbed, it represents a basic disruption of physiological stability. Even though sleep, in a purely technical sense, can be attained through the use of tranquilizers or other medications, we've seen that loss of consciousness by artificial means will not achieve balance in the body. In contrast, Ayurveda considers balance in an extremely comprehensive way, taking into account mind/body behavior as well as the environmental context.

In this regard, I would like to introduce a relaxation technique for creating tranquillity in your thoughts. You can use this technique when you're ready to go to bed or during the day when you feel the need to relax. It's a very simple but very powerful form of meditation.

I like to say that meditation is not at all a way of making your mind be quiet; rather, it's a way of entering into the quiet that's already there, buried under the fifty thousand thoughts an average person thinks every day. And, of course, most of those thoughts are really more than reflexes; they're automatic mental responses we've developed from conditioning that has filled us with anxiety and fear. They're nothing more than habits, and 99 percent of the thoughts you have today are the same ones you had the day before.

Yet all this mental static only masks the profound internal silence that is the real source of happiness, inspiration, and peace. Once you gain access to this silent realm of your mind, you achieve freedom from all those random images that trigger worry, anger, and pain.

Although you can use this technique anywhere, our present purpose here is to overcome insomnia and bring about good sleep. Therefore, when you use the technique, it's best to wait until you're in bed and ready to bring the day to a close. Let me emphasize that you should never undertake any sort of meditation while driving a car or operating any sort of machinery.

To begin, sit or lie down quietly with your hands lightly at your sides or folded in your lap. Then close your eyes, begin to breathe easily and naturally, and let your attention follow your breathing.

Feel your breath entering your nostrils and flowing down into your lungs. You don't need to inhale deeply or hold your breath, just breathe normally and easily. When you exhale, let your attention follow the air up out of your lungs and softly out through your nostrils.

Nothing needs to be forced. Just feel your breath moving

gently and easily, with your attention following it as naturally and effortlessly as a shadow.

Now, as your breathing relaxes, let it become a little lighter. Again, there's no need to force this, but when you feel that your breath is growing a bit shallower and lighter, simply let it happen. If you start to feel a bit short of breath, don't worry; however, this might mean that you're forcing your breathing to become lighter than it wants to be. So return naturally to whatever rate of breathing your body feels comfortable with.

Continue this exercise for two to five minutes, keeping your eyes closed and focusing your mind on easy, natural breathing.

When you've practiced this technique a few times, you'll begin to notice how, just by paying attention to your breathing, your body sinks deeper and deeper into relaxation, and your mind naturally becomes quieter, too. Before long you'll get a few glimpses of a profound and complete silence. You won't have to look for this silence; you'll just begin to lose track of your thoughts, and then the silence will simply appear.

As you gain experience with meditation, you'll of course begin to sleep better at night. But you'll also experience a kind of energy and vitality during the day that has its source at a deep level of the nervous system. This is a very profound change and an enormous benefit, and it could certainly never be brought about by medication.

DIET

Perhaps the main distinction between the modern nutritional understanding of diet and that of Ayurveda is that modern nutrition understands food only in terms of its material qualities.

To get an idea of what this means, consider the broad range of nutritional terminology that is used today: protein, carbohydrates, fats, minerals, cholesterol, vitamins, calories, and so forth. Each of these terms describes a particular material or chemical quality of food. Ayurveda, on the other hand, inter-prets the influence of food in terms of its intelligence value. Ayurveda recognizes the material value of the food, but it also explains that a more basic level of influence is derived from every form of nutrition. This influence is on the level of the mind/body connection. In other words, it is intelligence.

To understand what it really means to influence the physiol-ogy from this level, think of a tree with all its different elements: branches, bark, leaves, and fruits. It should be clear that the most effective way to influence the tree would not be to ap-proach each element—each leaf or branch or fruit—individu-ally. Instead, by bringing water to the tree, nature's intelligence is imparted to each and every one of its many aspects.

Similarly, your diet can influence your mind/body system in a very profound way. You've already learned the Ayurvedic ter-minology that can help you understand how to produce this in-fluence. You can understand, therefore, that every food will influence the physiology through the doshas, which in turn gov-ern the flow of nature's intelligence in the physiology.

Vata, of course, is the most important dosha in treating in-somnia. This is because Vata governs all movement, and excess Vata is responsible for the excessive mental activity or hyper-arousal that so commonly results in sleeplessness. The com-prehensive nutritional knowledge of Ayurveda ascribes to every substance and every food a particular influence on Vata, Pitta, and Kapha. For instance, certain foods are known to reduce Vata in the body. Eating these foods helps to transform the phys-iology so as to produce a more balanced state of functioning and a more settled awareness, and this in turn will alleviate in-somnia. While it's not necessary to stick to this Vata-pacifying diet very strictly, you should try to eat according to these prin-ciples:

1. It is very important to eat your meals regularly. As dis-cussed in the lesson on biological rhythms, taking meals at a set

time helps reset your body's biological clock. Remember that lunch is the time for the most important meal, and it should also be the heaviest meal of the day.

2. In general, favor warm, cooked, substantial meals. Balanced, solid meals, eaten on a regular schedule, will help soothe and settle the Vata dosha and make the body more comfortable at bedtime.

3. In describing nutrition, Ayurveda refers to six tastes: *sweet, sour, salty, pungent, bitter,* and *astringent.* The first three are those that most effectively pacify the Vata dosha. While a balanced diet will include all six tastes, these three should be emphasized. It's important to note that "sweet" does not mean just "sugary" but includes many wholesome foods such as milk, bread, grains, and pasta. Although the sweet taste is beneficial for Vata, concentrated sugar eaten by itself often gives a quick energy boost that can make Vata types feel very restless. If you eat a sugary sweet, take it along with something more nourishing, such as milk, which will balance the effect.

THE SIX TASTES AND EXAMPLES

Sweet	Sugar, milk, butter, rice, breads, pasta
Sour	Yogurt, lemons, cheese, vinegar, sour-tasting fruits
Salty	Salt
Pungent	Spicy foods, ginger, hot peppers, cumin, radishes
Bitter	Bitter greens (endive, chicory, romaine lettuce); other green, leafy vegetables; tonic water; turmeric; fenugreek
Astringent	Beans, lentils, pomegranates, cabbage, apples, potatoes, pears

HOW THE TASTES AFFECT THE DOSHAS

Decrease Vata	Sweet, sour, salty
Increase Vata	Pungent, bitter, astringent
Decrease Pitta	Sweet, bitter, astringent
Increase Pitta	Pungent, sour, salty
Decrease Kapha	Pungent, bitter, astringent
Increase Kapha	Sweet, sour, salty

VATA-PACIFYING DIET

Favor foods that are warm, heavy, and oily
Minimize foods that are cold, dry, and rough
Favor foods that are sweet, sour, and salty
Minimize foods that are spicy, bitter, and astringent

SPECIFIC RECOMMENDATIONS

- **Dairy.** All dairy products pacify Vata. Always boil milk before you drink it, and drink it warm. Don't drink milk with a full meal.
- **Sweeteners.** All sweeteners are good (in moderation) for pacifying Vata. However, concentrated sugar, when eaten by itself, can give a quick energy boost and make you feel extremely restless. If you eat a sugary sweet, try combining it with something more nourishing, like milk, to balance the effect. Raw, unrefined sugar, available in health food stores, is preferable to refined sugar.
- **Oils.** All oils are good, as they reduce Vata.
- **Grains.** Rice and wheat are very good. Reduce your intake of barley, corn, millet, buckwheat, rye, and oats.
- **Fruits.** Favor sweet, sour, or heavy fruits, such as oranges, bananas, avocados, grapes, cherries, peaches, melons, berries, plums, pineapples, mangoes, and papayas. Reduce astringent or light fruits, such as apples, pears, pomegranates, and cranberries.
- **Vegetables.** Beets, cucumbers, carrots, asparagus, and sweet potatoes are good. They should be eaten cooked, not raw. The following vegetables are acceptable in moderate quantities if they're cooked, especially with ghee or oil and Vata-reducing spices: peas; green, leafy vegetables; broccoli; cauliflower; celery; zucchini; and potatoes. It's better to avoid sprouts and cabbage.
- **Spices.** Cardamom, cumin, ginger, cinnamon, salt, cloves, mustard seed, and small quantities of black pepper are acceptable.
- **Nuts.** All nuts are good.
- **Beans.** Reduce all beans, except for tofu.
- **Meat and fish** (for nonvegetarians). Chicken, turkey, and seafoods are acceptable. Beef should be avoided.

Write down your favorite foods and spices from the **Vata-Pacifying Diet.** Then plan a few meals that include these foods. Record how you felt after eating these meals.

VATA PACIFYING FOODS AND SPICES I LIKE

1.	6.	11.
2.	7.	12.
3.	8.	13.
4.	9.	14.
5.	10.	15.

MEAL NUMBER ONE

MEAL NUMBER TWO

MEAL NUMBER THREE

Another useful tip for pacifying Vata is to avoid cold foods and drinks, especially those that are iced. This is because the Vata dosha is cold by nature, and anything cold will increase this effect. When you go out to dinner, ask for warm water to sip in place of ice water. Take the hot soup instead of the salad, and feel free to eat bread and butter as well as dessert, preferably a warm dessert like apple pie rather than ice cream, whose coldness will increase Vata in the system.

Remember that caffeine, cigarettes, and alcohol have been shown to interfere seriously with normal sleep. Alcohol eventually produces a state of drowsiness, of course, and can bring about loss of consciousness, but this is not natural sleep. The brain waves of people who drink alcohol show entirely different patterns from those of normal sleepers. For one thing, the dream stage of sleep is entirely bypassed. As a deficit of natural sleep builds up with continued alcohol use, there can be a very negative effect on general health.

This is especially true for a person in whom Vata has been disturbed. Even a single cup of tea or coffee, taken in the morning, can interfere with sleep that night. Don't forget that most soft drinks also contain caffeine, and that carbonated beverages in general will increase Vata and so should be minimized. Also, many prescriptions and over-the-counter medications contain stimulants. As we'll discuss in chapter 8, it is very common for people to experience sleep problems related to their medications. Consult your physician to determine whether this might apply to you.

Heavy food at dinner is not recommended. Although it may seem unusual, a hot breakfast cereal for dinner will taste extremely good to anyone suffering from a Vata imbalance. Other soothing, relatively light dinners are hearty minestrone soup, rice served with buttered lentils, or pasta in any form. Warm milk before bed is a good idea, but a late-night snack is not.

ELIMINATING IMPURITIES

Before leaving the subject of diet, I'd like to introduce a special technique for eliminating impurities or toxins from the system. In Ayurveda these impurities are called *amas*. Amas block normal functioning of the physiology and disturb the doshas. They are the residues of foods that have not been properly digested and that remain in the system in the form of toxins. Often they originate in greasy, stale, or heavy foods such as cheese or products made with white flour or refined sugar.

Sipping hot water during the day is an easy and effective way to dissolve ama and so eliminate it from the system. The concept is a simple one: Ama is described in Ayurvedic texts as a sticky white substance that clogs the channels of the physiology. When you wash dishes that are greasy or sticky, you use hot water to clean them; you can use hot water in the same way to remove ama gradually from your system.

While this method may sound remarkably simple, once you try drinking hot water you'll be impressed by the results. In addition to benefiting your sleep, your body will feel lighter and more energetic, and you'll experience a balanced mental awareness. But there is a specific routine that you must follow to produce this effect. First, the water should be very hot—so hot that you have to blow on it before you sip it. Second, the amount of hot water you take is less important than how frequently you take it. For best effect, the water should be sipped about every thirty minutes. If this seems too frequent for you, then take one or two sips of hot water every hour at the minimum. You can have much more if you like, according to your thirst.

You may also have other liquids during the day, but always take your hot water. The easiest way for most people to do this is to buy a good thermos and fill it in the morning with boiling water, which will remain hot for about ten hours. After a few days you will feel so soothed and balanced from this routine that you'll begin to look forward to it. You may find that for the first few weeks you urinate more frequently—and it may seem like even more than the amount by which you have increased your fluid intake. This is because the body is beginning to flush itself out to remove toxins and impurities from the system. It's a sign that something powerful is happening. After a few weeks the urine will return to normal, but the ama will continue to be eliminated from the system.

EXERCISE

Exercise is an important part of creating balance for any physiology. Cherak, one of the first Ayurvedic physicians, said the following: "From physical exercise, one gets lightness, capacity to work, firmness, tolerance of difficulties, diminution of physical impurities, and strengthening of digestion and metabolism."

While exercise is important for everyone, excessive exercise can be damaging. The three most common mistakes people make in relation to exercise are, first, taking too little exercise or none at all; second, performing exercises that don't suit their body type; and third, exercising beyond the point where risks begin to outweigh benefits. Therefore, the amount and type of exercise should be carefully suited to the individual. Above all, the purpose should be to produce energy and strength and vitality, not to use it up. You should feel lively, strong, and energetic during a workout and afterward. If you feel exhausted and strained at any point, then something is wrong with that particular program.

Sleep research shows inconsistent effects of exercise on sleep. Perhaps this is because the studies do not take into account the different body types of the individuals participating in the studies and the types of exercise they need. Of the three doshas, Kapha requires the most exercise. Vata requires the least, with Pitta in the middle.

Because insomnia is predominantly a Vata disorder, Ayurveda recommends only light to moderate exercise for those suffering from this problem—about thirty minutes per day of continuous motion. Brisk walking, cycling, swimming, and certain indoor exercises, such as stationary bicycling or a cross-country ski machine, are recommended. Always keep in mind the fact that excessive exercise can disturb Vata, and that too much exercise can be as harmful as too little.

If you're in the habit of vigorous exercise such as jogging five to ten miles at any time, try cutting back by half for one month and see what the effect is on your sleep. The Ayurvedic principle is to exercise to about 50 percent of your capacity. If you can bicycle twenty miles, do ten. If you usually run ten miles, run five. Your ultimate capacity is that point when you are completely tired and must stop, when you literally can't go any farther. Since what we want from exercise is not to spend all of our energy but rather to produce more of it, reaching the point of exhaustion should never be the goal. By stopping at about 50 percent, you should still feel energetic and comfortable, never strained or tired. In any case, the principle of utilizing half of your capacity does not violate the principles of physical conditioning. On the contrary. With regular exercise, your total capacity will increase, so that 50 percent of that capacity will also be increasing.

Integrating thirty minutes of walking once a day into your daily routine will have a profound effect in balancing the physiology and producing a more settled state of mind. The best time for exercise is during the Kapha period of morning, 6:00 to 10:00 A.M. On the other hand, exercising in the evening can aggravate insomnia by overstimulating the system too close to bedtime. In addition to walking, neuromuscular and neuro-respiratory integration exercises balance all three doshas simultaneously. These exercises, coming from the yoga tradition, not only benefit muscular and metabolic performance but enhance coordination between mind and body. Many people have found that neurorespiratory exercise, breathing exercise, produces a more settled state of awareness and is very useful for the treatment of insomnia.

PROPER EXERCISE

Exercise every day, using these Ayurvedic guidelines:

- Take a daily 30-minute walk. The best time is during the Kapha period in the morning, 6:00–10:00 A.M. Do not exercise (aside from easy walking) after 6:00 P.M.
- You can substitute other light to moderate exercises of a continuous motion, such as cycling and swimming. Using a stationary bicycle or cross-country ski machine is also recommended.
- Use only 50 percent of your capacity. For example, if you can cycle six miles, cycle three. If you are capable of swimming eight laps, stop after four. With regular exercise, your capacity will grow.
- Do not strain. You should feel strong and energetic during and after exercise.
- If you are in the habit of exercising vigorously, try cutting back by half for one month and see what effect this change has on your sleep.

Do the following Neuromuscular and Neurorespiratory Integration Exercises for a few minutes daily. If possible, do them twice a day before you meditate. The best times are in the morning after bathing and in the evening before supper.

NEUROMUSCULAR INTEGRATION EXERCISES

These simple exercises, or yoga postures, help restore mind/body coordination and balance all levels of your body's functioning.

Guidelines to Follow

1. Be careful not to strain by stretching too far. The drawings show the **ideal** performance of each exercise, but

should stretch only as far as your body is comfortable. Over time you will develop more flexibility. You should definitely avoid stretching to the point of pain or discomfort.

If even minimal performance of a particular posture causes pain or discomfort, omit that posture. If you have a chronic or acute muscular or skeletal condition (back problem), consult your physician before doing these exercises.

2. If you feel that you cannot bend a particular part of your body, don't force your body by swinging. Just bend to the extent you can, without trying to force.

3. Hold each posture for only a few seconds and then release it easily. Just breathe naturally during the exercises—do not hold your breath.

4. Wear comfortable, loose clothing. Use a folded wool blanket, rug, or exercise mat rather than the bare floor.

5. Do not perform the postures on a full stomach. This means you should wait at least two or three hours after a meal before doing these exercises.

6. When you are performing these postures, easily allow your attention to focus on the area of your body that is being stretched. By doing the postures in quiet and without disturbance, your attention will automatically be drawn to that area of your body. Just by allowing your awareness to be on the area of maximum stretch, you will gain the maximum benefit from the exercise.

7. These exercises take only about five minutes if you perform each posture once. If you have time, you can repeat each exercise three times.

8. Be sure to follow the sequence of poses given below, as each pose is designed to prepare your body for the next one.

1   TONING-UP EXERCISES

This two-minute body massage gently increases circulation, moving your blood in the direction of your heart.

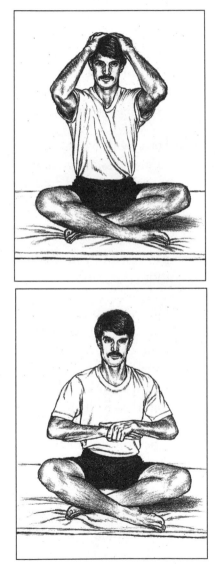

1. Sit comfortably. Use the palms and fingers of both hands to press the top of your head, gradually moving them toward your face, neck, and chest while pressing and releasing. Then start again at the top of your head and gradually press and release down over the back of your neck and around to your chest.

2. Grasp the fingertips of your right hand with the palm and fingers of your left hand, gradually pressing and releasing your arm up to your shoulder and chest. First do the upper side of your arm, then repeat on the underside. Then massage your left arm in the same way.

3. With the tips of your fingers meeting horizontally at the navel, begin to press and release your abdomen, gradually moving the pressure up toward your heart, reaching almost to your chest.

4. Use both hands to press and release the middle of your back and ribs up toward your heart as far as you can reach.

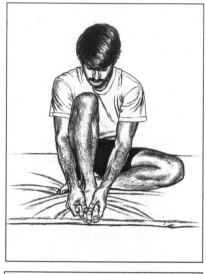

5. Start with your right foot, massaging your toes and sole and gradually pressing and releasing up your calf, thigh, and waist. Repeat with your left foot.

6. Lie on your back, draw your knees up to your chest, and clasp your hands over your knees. Raise your head slightly. Roll to the right until your right wrist touches the floor, then roll to the left. Repeat five times in each direction, then slowly stretch your legs out until you are lying on your back. Rest for a few seconds.

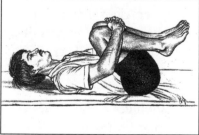

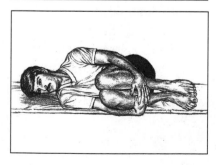

2   SEAT-STRENGTHENING POSE

This exercise prepares your body for the other postures, strengthening your pelvic area and back.

1. Kneel down, sitting on the flats of your feet, with heels apart and your big toes crossed. Place your hands in your lap, palms up. Hold your head, neck, and spine in a straight line.

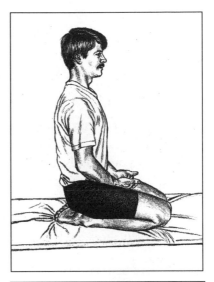

2. Next, lift your buttocks off your heels until you are in a kneeling position. Then slowly lower your body and sit down on your heels again. Repeat, moving slowly and smoothly.

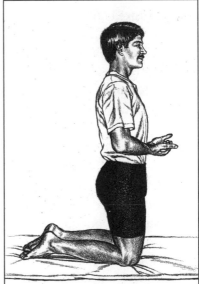

3   HEAD-TO-KNEE POSE

This posture strengthens and relaxes your spine and abdominal organs, aiding in digestion.

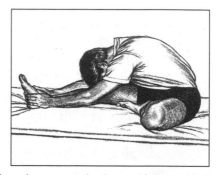

1. Sit and stretch your right leg in front of you. Bend your left leg so the sole of your foot is touching the inside of your thigh.
2. Bend forward and touch your right foot with your hands, arms outstretched. You can bend your right knee if you need to. Hold the pose for a few seconds, then slowly release it and come up to a sitting position.
3. Repeat the exercise, using your other leg.

4   SHOULDER STAND

This posture enlivens the endocrine system and the thyroid gland, relieves mental fatigue, makes your spine more flexible, and has a soothing effect on your body.

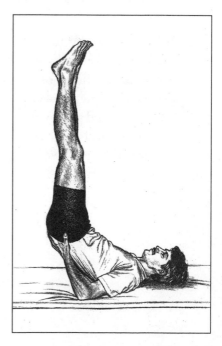

1. Lie on your back. Slowly raise your legs to a half-vertical position, over the waist. Support your back with your hands above your hips, keeping your elbows in toward your body.

2. Tilt your feet more toward your head. Hold the pose for half a minute.

3. Slowly return to the original position by bending your knees to balance your trunk until your buttocks touch the floor, then straighten your legs and lower them slowly. Relax gradually. Breathe normally and naturally throughout all the exercises.

4. Be careful not to strain your neck or throat—this is a shoulder stand, not a neck stand.

5   PLOW POSE

This pose strengthens and relaxes your back, neck, and shoulders. It normalizes the functioning of the liver, spleen, and thyroid and removes fatigue.

1. From the shoulder stand, continue into this position as you bend from your pelvis and bring both legs down over your head.

2. Allow your legs to go back only as far as feels comfortable. Be careful not to put too much strain on your neck. Extend your arms straight out behind you. Your torso should rest on the tops of your shoulders, your hips maintaining a vertical line with your shoulder joints. Cross your arms over your head, holding for a few seconds.

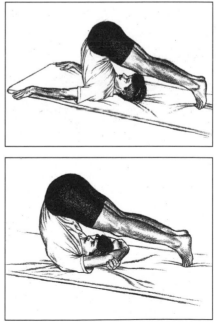

3. Slowly return to a prone position by bending your knees to balance your torso until your buttocks touch the floor. Then straighten your legs and lower them slowly. Relax.

6   COBRA POSE

This exercise strengthens and relaxes your back muscles and helps with irregularities in the ovaries and uterus.

1. Lie on your chest with your palms directly under your shoulders, fingers pointing forward. Place your forehead on the floor.
2. Slowly raise your head and chest, keeping your elbows close in to your body, and maintain the pose for a few seconds.
3. Bend your elbows, slowly lowering yourself until you are lying comfortably, resting your right or left cheek on the floor. Relax completely.

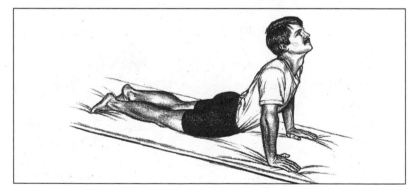

7   LOCUST POSE

This posture strengthens your lower back, aids in digestion, and balances the bladder, prostate, uterus, and ovaries.

1. Continue to lie on your chest, with your arms along the sides of your body, palms up. Let your chin rest gently on the floor.

2. Raise your legs in a straight position, extending them upward and back. Hold the pose for a few seconds while breathing easily. Then release your legs slowly.

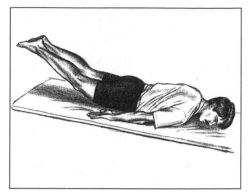

3. If you find it difficult to raise both legs together in the beginning, do not strain. Try raising one leg at a time.

8 SEATED TWIST POSE

This pose increases circulation in the liver, spleen, adrenal glands, and kidneys. It also releases tightness in the shoulders, upper back, and neck.

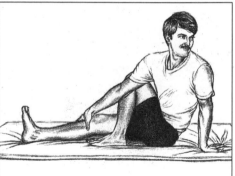

1. Sit with your legs stretched out in front of you.
2. Raise your left leg so that your foot is on the floor near your right knee.
3. Put your left hand on the floor behind you.
4. Gently turn your torso to the left, press your right forearm against the outside of your left knee, and grasp your right leg below the knee.
5. Turn your head and torso to your left.
6. Maintain the pose for a few seconds and come back slowly to the original seated position. Repeat the pose with your other leg.

9   STANDING FORWARD BEND

This exercise strengthens internal functioning of the liver, stomach, spleen, and kidneys. It tones the spine and soothes and relaxes the mind.

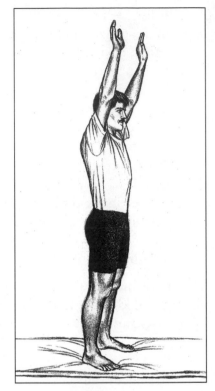

1. Stand up straight with your feet parallel, about as wide apart as your hips. Stand with your weight distributed evenly on both feet.

2. Bend forward until your hands touch your toes (or as far as is comfortable). Stretch your arms and allow your forehead to either touch your knees or be near them. Notice that your abdomen is naturally drawn in during this pose.

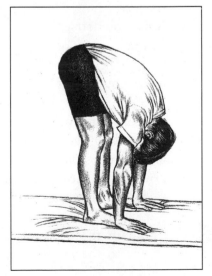

10   AWARENESS POSE

This soothing pose eliminates fatigue and rejuvenates the body and mind.

1. Lie on your back, allowing your arms to rest easily by your sides with your palms up.
2. Allow your body to relax. Close your eyes and let your awareness be easily drawn to any part of your body or to your body as a whole.
3. Rest for at least one minute, breathing easily and naturally.

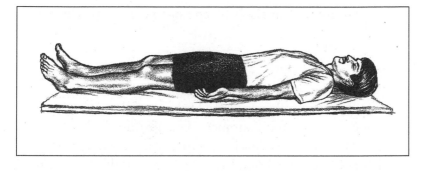

NEURORESPIRATORY INTEGRATION EXERCISE

This simple exercise, called Pranayama, creates balance throughout your body. It helps settle your awareness, which is especially useful in treating insomnia. It's ideal to do Pranayama after the Neuromuscular Integration Exercises.

How to Do Pranayama

1. Sit easily and comfortably with your spine as straight as possible.
2. Close your eyes and rest your **left** hand on your knees or thighs. For this exercise you will be using your thumb and the middle and ring fingers of your **right** hand.

3. Using your right thumb, close off your right nostril. Start by exhaling through your left nostril. Then inhale easily through your left nostril.

4. Now use your ring and middle fingers to close your left nostril. Exhale slowly through your right nostril, then easily inhale.

5. Continue alternating nostrils for about five minutes. Your breathing should be natural, not exaggerated. It may be a little slower and deeper than usual.

6. When you are finished, sit quietly with your eyes closed for a few minutes while breathing easily and normally.

Continue using your **Daily Sleep Log** and **Bedtime Checklist**.

HERBS

Thousands of naturally occurring herbs are utilized in Ayurveda and are considered food supplements. Just as food influences physiology at the basic level of nature's intelligence, herbs are also beneficial on this level, but they can be utilized more precisely to influence a particular aspect of Vata, Pitta, or Kapha doshas. With regard to insomnia, herbal supplements are used as part of an overall strategy that includes creating balance in the physiology at all levels—body, mind, and spirit. Ayurveda considers the following herbs in various combinations particularly useful for treating insomnia. These combinations are available through the Ayurvedic resources whose addresses are provided at the back of this book.

The herbs, along with some of their properties, are:

- Jatamamsi, a close relative of tagara, which creates cooling energy and aids digestion
- Ashwagandha, rejuvenating herb, which calms the nerves and promotes satisfying rest

- Shakhanalpushpi, another herb which strengthens the nervous system and calms the mind
- Brahmi, which is useful for pacifying Pitta as well as Vata
- Jatiphala, one of the best herbs for treating the nervous disorders that can disrupt sleep
- Tagara, whose Latin name is *valerian*, especially useful for cleansing accumulated Vata from the nervous system. The usefulness of valerian as a sleep aid has been confirmed by Western medicine in a study conducted in Switzerland. Among 128 subjects, the herb did improve sleep and there were no measurable side effects.

Although the herbs listed above are naturally occurring substances that have been used for thousands of years in many societies, any preparation can cause an unwanted reaction in some individuals. If you're interested in using herbs to help you sleep, be sure to do so with the guidance of experienced Ayurvedic teachers, some of whom can be contacted through the addresses provided at the end of this book.

Some of the points covered in this chapter may seem related less to insomnia than to altering your bedtime, but remember that Ayurveda's approach is both comprehensive and unique. It is an extremely thorough process that allows you to simultaneously balance mind, body, behavior, and environment. You'll be surprised at the effects that these additional routines will have in enhancing your well-being; they will help not only in overcoming insomnia but in all areas of your life.

7

DREAMS AND DREAMING

Dreaming, like sleep itself, is a highly subjective phenomenon that has been interpreted in contradictory ways during different historical periods, in different societies, and by different individuals. Until quite recently, however, it seemed there was one thing that everyone agreed about—that *dreams are important*.

From ancient times, when biblical characters like Joseph or Daniel could ascend to high position based on their ability to interpret dreams, to Freud, whose revolutionary book *The Interpretation of Dreams* was published in 1900, there has been a sense that dreams are occurrences we can learn from. At first it was believed that dreams could tell us about the future of an entire society—whether there would be famine, for instance, or whether an invasion was coming. More recently, the importance of dreams was seen in more concentrated terms: If dreams could no longer tell us about the world at large, they could still reveal important truths about the individual dreamer.

I personally believe that dreams are important, or at least

some of them are. Aside from the issue of interpretation, there's no doubt that certain dreams, such as nightmares, can influence how you feel and how you behave the following day. It's also true that certain happy dreams can allow you to start the day feeling particularly well; some can even cause you to wake up laughing. Quite as much as the actual amount of time spent sleeping, dreams can mean the difference between a good night's sleep and a bad one.

Let's now consider some of the more interesting and enigmatic qualities of dreams, especially those qualities that seem related to insomnia. We'll also see how modern scientific methods, as well as the tradition of Ayurveda, have understood these dream characteristics.

PARABLES AND PARADOXES

As discussed earlier, the purpose of sleep is to rest and restore the physiology. Like a rechargeable battery, the sleeping body goes into a sort of diminished state of functioning for a period of time that allows it to regain the energy that was used up during the hours when it was "on."

This model of the recharging battery makes perfect sense when applied to many of the bodily functions—except during the REM (rapid eye movement) period of sleep, which is when dreaming occurs, and which lasts about two hours during a normal night's sleep. For most of our sleep time, such measures as heart rate, breathing rate, and blood pressure are lowered. But with the onset of REM, metabolism reaches a higher rate, the kidneys begin working harder, and, in men, the penis becomes erect. With respect to the brain, the metaphor of the battery begins to grow even dimmer. That is because in some important respects—blood flow to the brain, for example—the dreaming brain is even more active than the waking one.

According to Dr. William C. Dement, a leading sleep researcher at Stanford University, it makes perfect sense that the brain is so busy during the REM period. The dreaming brain is, after all, doing everything it does during waking hours, and even more. During waking hours the brain needs only to respond to a preexisting external reality, and then to implement the appropriate physiological responses. These responses can take the form of bodily movements, spoken words, or thoughts. The dreaming brain, on the other hand, has to *create* an entire internal reality, as well as respond to it.

If, for example, a runaway horse is charging toward you during your waking hours, your brain will receive a message that the horse is coming, and it will respond by sending a message to your legs to take you out of the way. But when a horse charges toward you in a dream, your brain has had to create that horse, not just receive a message about it. Furthermore, the neural response that your dreaming brain sends to your legs is every bit as highly developed as it would be if you were awake. The response message travels through your nervous system all the way to your legs, only to be neutralized at the last instant by the unique bodily paralysis that characterizes the REM period. The impulse to run away turns into, at the very most, a barely perceptible twitch of a muscle—but that isn't because the brain didn't try its hardest.

Remember: Nature doesn't do anything for nothing. If the purpose of sleep is indeed to restore the body, we must account for the fact that during a significant portion of our sleep time this restoration isn't accomplished simply through passive rest. Instead, a positive, active process is taking place that requires significant energy.

This seems a paradox. How can the energy expenditure be justified in the cause of rest? Why doesn't nature, which we've described as always taking the path of least resistance, simply take the easy way out and shut everything down all night long?

There must be some way to account for the physiological work that's required to create all the animals, answering machines, and antique stores that comprise the parables of our dreams. Any number of solutions have been proposed to explain. Unfortunately, they don't lead to any single overwhelming conclusion, but are instead as paradoxical as dreams themselves.

TO REMEMBER, OR TO FORGET?

One of the most hazardous concepts in scientific thinking is known as the *Ptolemaic fallacy*. This term is derived from the description of the universe according to the ancient astronomer Ptolemy, whose work accurately accounted for the observable phenomena, but was in fact wrong. In other words, the sun *seems* to be rotating around the Earth, and you can develop a whole cosmology based on that appearance. But the sun isn't rotating around the Earth, regardless of how it seems.

With respect to the purpose of dreams, there are many approaches that seem to account for what is taking place, but in reality they may be accurate representations of nothing except the creativity of the investigator. That doesn't mean they don't seem convincing, however. It is easy for an extremely intelligent person, especially a scientist, to build an argument that can convince a layperson or even the public at large. In the eighteenth-century novel *Rasselas*, by Samuel Johnson, a scientist explains a set of mechanical wings he's invented which will allow people to fly like birds. His argument is beautifully wrought and extremely convincing, even to the modern reader. It's very difficult to find anything wrong with it. Of course, when the character jumps off a roof, the elegance of his reasoning doesn't help him.

Sigmund Freud, the founder of psychoanalysis, thought that dreams were a way of processing wishes that could not safely be acted out in the waking world. Instead, they're acted out in the dreaming world, with the body paralyzed and unable to get into any trouble. But does anyone really wish to have a horse come charging at him, as in the dream I mentioned above? Perhaps not—but the dream is only a disguised form of the repressed wish. If the wish were dreamed in a too straightforward fashion, the dreamer would awaken in fear of the productions of his own brain, and the biological benefits of sleep would be lost. In fact, according to Freud, this is exactly what happens in nightmares.

So Freud sees dreams as a sort of compromised version of fulfilling wishes that are unacceptable to the conscious mind, under the need of the body to get the rest that sleep provides.

Freud's thinking has been of monumental influence throughout this century, of course. Even those more recent investigators who disagree with his conclusions (as most of them do) find themselves having to deal with the issues that Freud raised, and even use some of his terminology.

For example, studies of sleeping cats by researchers at Harvard University revealed that bursts of brain activity occur at intervals during REM sleep. These "brainstorms" flood the neural pathways. Believing that similar bursts of activity occur in humans, the researchers infer that it's the task of the sleeping human brain to deal with these sudden floods of random sensory data. In order to do so, the brain does its best to create a story that weaves everything together. The brain naturally draws upon the dreamer's wishes and fears in order to accomplish this, as in the Freudian theory, but repression has no place in the brainstorm doctrine. Far from trying to hide anything, the brain is looking for whatever it can find to help make sense of the data.

In a related theory, the sleeping brain is again described as weaving together a large amount of raw data, but instead of originating as sudden neural bursts from inside itself, the random material now derives from the events of the previous day in the waking world, with all its comings and goings, conversations, and so forth. During REM sleep, the brain creates a story line that allows this large volume of events to be stored and remembered in a coherent form, albeit at an unconscious level. According to this theory, the dream is an elaborate mnemonic device for the events of your life. A dream is really a memory aid.

Or perhaps the purpose of dreams is to help us *forget*. Research by the eminent Francis Crick, one of the discoverers of the structure of the DNA molecule, concludes that the neural bursts that occur during REM are really a form of cleansing the system. The brain is simply dumping its electrical garbage. This approach has an undeniable logic in its favor. After all, we usually don't remember our dreams, so it must not have been nature's intention that we should do so.

THE AYURVEDIC APPROACH

Ayurveda is above all a practical system. Since dreams have a less direct influence on health and well-being than issues such as digestion or nutrition, Ayurvedic authorities had less to say about them than did other, more mystical traditions. But Ayurveda does offer a number of insights about dreams and dreamers.

As in waking life, the key influence on an individual's dreams is his or her body type.

Vata types typically have very imaginative dreams that are colored by fear or anxiety. This tendency becomes more pronounced as the dosha goes out of balance—so if you are a Vata type and you notice your dreams becoming more intense, you should take steps to restore stability. Of course, even if this is not your primary dosha, you can have frightening dreams when your Vata is unbalanced. In Ayurveda, such dreams are understood as a natural correction, your body's way of getting disturbed Vata back into balance. We'll deal more specifically with this in a moment, when we discuss nightmares.

Pitta types have active, adventurous dreams, often characterized by angry or conflicting situations such as fights or mysteries. It's interesting to note that dream research shows these themes to be primarily male characteristics. Women's dreams typically feature more conversation than hard action. Women's dreams also tend to be set in interior locations more than men's.

Kapha types have serene dreams that are usually not recalled. It's possible that Kaphas, who are typically very deep, sound sleepers, spend more time in the dreamless, delta phase of sleep than in the REM phase.

NIGHTMARES: WHEN SLEEP IS WORSE THAN BEING AWAKE

One of the reasons I think dreams are important is that they've had a profound influence on our cultural heritage. For instance, it's very difficult to imagine what Western literature would be like if human beings didn't dream. For example, in the works of Shakespeare, *Hamlet*, *Macbeth*, *Richard III*, and a number of other plays would have to be fundamentally different. This central importance of dreams is true for Oriental literature as well.

But it's not just dreams that are important to the history of the human imagination—it's *nightmares* that are important. The paintings of Goya and Fuseli, the novels of Dostoyevsky and Kafka, and the music of Schoenberg come to mind as being explicitly influenced by the experience of anxiety-laden dreams.

And for our purposes here, nightmares are significant as well. Because while they may foster the creation of a great work of art, they can most definitely wreck a good night's sleep.

Sleep research has revealed a number of characteristics by which nightmares can be defined:

- A nightmare causes the sleeper to awaken from REM usually in a state of fear but without physical symptoms such

as rapid pulse or sweating. These in turn are characteristic of "sleep terrors," which occur during delta sleep.
- Nightmares are often recalled in their entirety by the dreamer, and often in great detail.
- Frequently, people who suffer from nightmares can recognize recurring themes, and sometimes a whole dream repeats itself many times, occasionally for many years.

Considered by themselves, nightmares are not an especially important cause of insomnia: approximately 5 percent of the adult American population is bothered by them at any given time. Nightmares may, however, be a symptom of other, more basic issues. For example, a high percentage of chronic nightmare sufferers have experienced a traumatic event or period in their lives that has remained unresolved, perhaps even unrecognized. Another large segment of the nightmare-troubled population have had these dreams since childhood, often for reasons that contemporary medicine is unable to identify—although an Ayurvredic diagnosis would most likely be able to identify the cause in a dosha imbalance. I will have more to say about this in the next chapter, when we discuss the problem of childhood-onset insomnia.

If your insomnia is caused or exacerbated by nightmares, the best course is probably what we've been saying all along: You must look to your waking life to understand what's happening to your sleep. Many nightmares don't have a deep underlying cause. There may be tension at work or within your family. Clinical experience shows that once this is identified and dealt with, the troubling dreams disappear. It's as simple as that.

While it used to be said that eating certain foods shortly before bed could cause nightmares, this has not been demonstrated in any rigorously structured studies. There is no doubt, however, that nightmares can be brought on by taking the wrong medication, and especially by drinking too much alcohol. Once again, the solution is quite simple.

8

INSOMNIA IN CHILDREN

AND IN THE ELDERLY

Balance and moderation are the keystones of the Ayurvedic approach to health, and this applies to sleeping habits as well. There's an interesting piece of research that demonstrates the wisdom of this viewpoint. The American Cancer Society questioned a random sample of adults about their sleep patterns, then ran a follow-up study six years later. The results showed that 99 percent of the subjects who averaged between seven and nine hours per night were still alive. But the death rate of those who slept more than ten hours per night was almost double that of the "normal" sleepers—and for men who slept fewer than four hours a night, the mortality rate was almost 300 percent higher.

This study doesn't prove that sleeping too much or too little can cause premature death, but it strongly suggests a correlation. It might have been useful to know more about the people who were at the opposite ends of the scale. What were their lifestyles and habits? What kinds of work did they do? And most important, what were their ages. There's strong evidence that age is the most important factor in determining an individual's sleep pattern. This is the view of modern science, and this is also the Ayurvedic view.

According to Ayurveda, childhood is dominated by the Kapha dosha, and that's when we all tend to sleep the longest. Newborns sometimes sleep almost the entire day immediately after birth; the average baby sleeps about sixteen hours on that day, and for weeks afterward as well. Even at the age of 5, children should have almost twelve hours of sleep daily. But by old age, which is a Vata period of life, sleep time for the average person has typically declined to five or six hours, even in people who slept longer in their middle years.

Insomnia in both childhood and old age tends to be a more serious problem than the kind of "situational" insomnia encountered by people in their middle years, where the cause is often relatively easy to identify and adjust. In this chapter, therefore, we'll look at some of the special characteristics of insomnia among the very young and the elderly.

CHILDHOOD-ONSET INSOMNIA

For most children, sleep is a simple, natural response to an internal signal. As soon as children are sufficiently tired, they go to sleep. Sometimes that signal may not be heard as promptly as parents would like, but when it is heard, it's heeded, and the child falls asleep.

Unfortunately, this is not the case with all children. A small percentage experience childhood-onset insomnia, which begins virtually at birth and continues into adult life. This is a serious problem that can have a profound impact on an individual's ability to enjoy life, and it often requires more aggressive treatment than other forms of insomnia.

Dr. Peter Hauri of the Mayo Clinic Insomnia Research Program has done intensive research into childhood-onset insomnia, both in its early stages and in adults who continue to experience sleep problems. Hauri found that insomnia in children is often accompanied by certain specific neurological problems, such as dyslexia and hyperactivity. (From an Ayurvedic point of view, it's significant that there's also a hypersensitivity to noise, which indicates unbalanced Vata.) Although dyslexia and hyperactivity are not necessarily indications of a psychological disorder, children experiencing them do respond positively to low dosages of antidepressant medications. These same medications can also relieve the symptoms of childhood insomnia.

Interestingly, very young victims of sleeplessness are far from depressed. On the contrary, they're exceedingly alert, exceptionally curious about the world around them, and ready for action at all times. For many years this kind of behavior in children was misunderstood as completely positive in character. But as the child grows older and begins to encounter responsibilities that place greater strain on the physiology, the inability to sleep well soon begins to take a toll. Adult victims of childhood-onset insomnia are often unable to hold a job or even to behave normally in everyday social interactions. Every day, they literally feel as a normal person would after participating in a sleep-deprivation experiment lasting hundreds of hours.

Fortunately, in addition to the antidepressant medications that are effective with children, there are other drugs that can help adults overcome their lifelong insomnia. But the same medicines don't work for everyone, and those that do work are often not at all what a physician might have expected. In other words, treatment is often a process of trial and error, but it can be successful under proper professional supervision.

If you've been troubled by extreme insomnia since early childhood and it has had a debilitating effect on your life, I strongly recommend that you seek treatment as soon as possible.

SLEEPWALKING AND CHILDREN'S NIGHTMARES

The peculiar phenomenon of sleepwalking is rarely encountered except in children, who almost always outgrow it by adolescence. Statistically, boys are much more likely to experience it than girls. The cause seems to be a genetic factor, since almost all sleepwalkers have relatives who displayed the same behavior at a similar age. Medication and psychotherapy are not of great benefit in this case, especially in children, so the best course is to let time solve the problem. Meanwhile, be sure to create a sleepwalking-safe environment. Windows should be locked, car keys should be hidden, and the sleepwalker's bedroom should be on the first floor.

Like "sleep terrors"—during which the subject awakens not only frightened but with physical symptoms such as rapid heartbeat—sleepwalking takes place during the deep, delta phase of sleep. Sleepwalkers are capable of performing simple tasks such as opening doors, but they are unable to drive cars or operate computers—which doesn't mean they won't try. They usually seem indifferent to their surroundings, as evidenced by their willingness to walk barefoot through snow.

What should you do if you encounter a sleepwalker? Folk medicine claims that psychological disaster will result if the walker is awakened. This is not correct in the scientific sense, but it can be frightening for the sleepwalker to abruptly find him- or herself in a very different setting from the bedroom. In any case, expert opinion suggests there's usually no need to awaken the walker, who can simply be taken gently by the arm and led back to bed.

About 15 percent of American children sleepwalk at least once in their lives. In contrast, virtually all children experience nightmares, and these obviously require compassion and reassurance from parents. Childhood nightmares occur most often between the ages of 3 and 8. In a typical sequence, the child wakes up in terror, finds him- or herself alone in a dark room, cries out, and then seeks refuge in bed with the parents.

There's nothing wrong with allowing this scenario to continue to its conclusion, with parents and child sleeping together, but that does nothing to break the chain of events that comprise the problem. A more proactive solution would be to deal with the terrifying environment of the child's dark room, which is as much a part of the nightmare experience as is the dream itself.

If possible, go to the room before the child gets out of bed and provide reassurances that the thing hanging on the chair is just a coat, not a werewolf. Do your best to persuade the child to remain in the room, and be willing to stay there yourself as long as necessary.

If this is a recurring problem, look for long-term solutions, which may be as simple as a night-light or an open door to the hall. According to many authorities, however, the best answer to children's nightmares is a family pet with whom to share the child's bedroom: The effectiveness of this approaches 100 percent. If keeping a live pet is impossible, a stuffed one is an alternative—but keep in mind that to the child, it may look like a werewolf in the dark.

SLEEP AND OLDER PEOPLE

In general, sleep disturbances become more frequent and more troublesome as we age. The body becomes more Vata after the age of 40, so older people often sleep very badly because Vata disturbances that haven't been treated only get worse.

Even more so than with other age groups, older people should remember that the key to sleeping well at night is to have an active day. If you're tired in a healthy way, your body can use the night to restore physiological balance by itself, without any need for drugs. Older people are often taking a wide variety of medications, but drugs of every sort impair good sleep, even if they seem to help in the short run. So medications should be kept to a minimum, sleeping pills should be avoided, and alcohol should be taken only in moderation.

As an individual ages, the body's excretory functions often become less efficient, which means that drugs can linger longer in the body. Whatever goes in takes longer to go out. Yet tests of sleeping pills and other medications are generally carried out on relatively young, healthy experimental subjects. Furthermore, these tests are usually carried out by the manufacturers of the medications themselves. For these reasons, a strong argument can be made that elderly people should take significantly less than the recommended dosages. As you'll see when we discuss the hugely underestimated problem of sleep apnea, elderly people manifest a close relationship between depression, so-called senility, and insomnia. Yet many studies have shown that when sleeping pills and other medications are reduced or withdrawn, the "senility" dramatically improves.

If an older person feels the need to take something to foster sleep, the best choice is warm milk with a spoonful of honey at bedtime, which is very soothing to Vata. It's also a good idea to drink plenty of water. While that might not seem like the most exciting thing in the world, dehydration is a major health concern for the elderly.

Remember too that Vata is extremely sensitive to loud noises and bright lights. These tendencies will naturally become stronger with age, particularly if someone is a Vata type to begin with. So the bedroom should be made as dark and quiet as possible. Sometimes, even without your being consciously aware of it, light coming in between curtains or under a door can trigger a waking response during the Vata period in the early morning.

SLEEP APNEA

The most serious and widespread of all sleep-related disorders is called *sleep apnea*, a medical term that refers to loss of respiration during sleep. Studies suggest that 25 percent of all Americans over age 65 are affected by this problem, which can be a precipitating factor of major depression, cardiovascular disease, and death.

Basically, sleep apnea causes the subject's breathing to cease for periods of up to sixty seconds during sleep, after which he or she wakes up gasping or coughing, remains awake or partially awake for only a second or two, usually without even opening the eyes, and then falls back to sleep, only to repeat the process. Since this sequence can occur as many as a thousand times during a single night, it's hardly surprising that the subject doesn't feel very well rested in the morning. Sleep apnea victims are rarely aware of the actual number of times they awakened, so their feelings of exhaustion, extreme drowsiness, and impaired thinking processes seem without explanation. But the real cause is extreme sleep deprivation.

Although this condition can occur in children, most victims are in their later years. There can be malformations or deterioration within the nasal breathing passages that contribute to the problem, but the most prominent indicators are overweight, alcohol consumption, and snoring. Literally all sleep apnea sufferers snore, and their spouses frequently report that snoring is worse after a nightcap or two.

Surgical procedures can repair many of the physiological problems that underlie sleep apnea. In many cases surgery is well justified, since a large percentage of the degenerative symptoms we associate with aging are in fact rooted in the inability of the subject to get a good night's rest. This is especially true for what's commonly referred to as senility, with its confused thinking, moodiness, and apathetic behavior. But there are many positive steps that can be taken before even considering surgery, the first of which must be an accurate assessment of the problem.

Since the typical sleep apnea patient thinks he or she awakens four or five times each night—when the actual number of mini-awakenings is perhaps a hundred times that—no one can expect to diagnose this condition alone. According to Dr. William Dement of Stanford University, everyone over the age of 65 should be evaluated for breathing disorders during sleep. This is especially true for people who snore, who are overweight, who are in the habit of taking alcohol in order to sleep, and who display signs of drowsiness throughout the day.

If allowed to persist, sleep apnea can cause hypertension and diminished levels of oxygen in the blood. In turn, these can bring on congestive heart failure, a leading cause of death among the elderly. In short, it's impossible for an older person to be considered emotionally or physically healthy if he or she isn't getting enough sleep as a result of sleep apnea.

FULFILLMENT, THE BASIS

FOR RESTFUL SLEEP

Just as light brightens darkness, discovering inner fulfillment can eliminate any disorder or discomfort, including insomnia. This is truly the key to creating balance and harmony in everything you do.

This chapter offers ideas and recommendations for increasing your sense of fulfillment and freeing your inner nature. After all, the goal of Ayurveda is to help you realize that you are made of pure awareness, that it is your natural state to be free from illness and fear, and that it is your destiny to enjoy complete fulfillment in life.

In presenting solutions to the problem of insomnia, it's essential to discuss the concept of personal fulfillment. Because with any health problem, Ayurveda takes a dual approach: It considers the specific physical imbalances that have come to exist, and on a different level, Ayurveda introduces a new element into the situation, and this is the element of fulfillment.

Several years ago, the Massachusetts Department of Health,

Education, and Welfare undertook a study of risk factors for heart disease. Hearing of this, you might ask if such a study was necessary. Why is anyone still looking at risk factors for heart disease? We know what they are: hypertension, smoking, cholesterol, family history, and so on. But actually there is still good reason to study cardiac risk factors, because the majority of people who have their first heart attack before the age of 50 do not display *any* of the so-called danger signals. In fact, the Massachusetts survey revealed that the real number-one risk factor for heart disease is job dissatisfaction—and the number-two risk factor for heart disease is a low sense of personal happiness.

That means you could go out on the street and ask people just two questions: Do you love your job? and, Are you really happy? If a person can comfortably answer yes to both these questions, he or she is probably going to avoid heart trouble and most other health problems as well, because risk for most illnesses concerns these two basic issues.

There is a concept in Ayurveda known as *dharma*. To be in dharma means to know what you're here for. It means you've discovered the purpose of your life. You see, there are no extra pieces in the universe. Everyone is here because he or she has a place to fill, and every piece must fit itself into the big jigsaw puzzle. Indeed, the universe would be incomplete if it weren't for the fact that you happen to be here. And for any single thing to happen in this whole universe, you and everyone else must take part in it.

Of course the concept of dharma encompasses much more than just job satisfaction. Dharma takes in all the activities of our waking state of consciousness, because we are destined to fulfillment, and part of that destiny is doing that work which gives us the most satisfaction.

But sometimes things can get in the way of our destiny. Insomnia, in fact, is one of the earlier problems that we might encounter, and it can be a harbinger of other problems. In Ayurveda, the source of any difficulty is said to lie in awareness. An awareness of some discomfort, some disease, some anxiety, some worry, which then becomes a background condition such as fatigue and insomnia. Next a sharper level of physical discomfort begins, and ultimately the full-blown expression of physical disease presents itself.

So insomnia is a symptom of an underlying imbalance, and if you want to discover the root cause of that imbalance, I would suggest it is lack of dharma, lack of fulfillment, lack of purpose in life.

To put it a better way, the purpose is there, but you haven't found it yet.

ASK THE BASIC QUESTIONS

To overcome any sleep-related difficulty, it's very important to implement the practical suggestions made in the earlier chapters of this book. But even as you're doing that, it's essential to ask yourself some very basic questions about your life: *What is my purpose here? . . . What makes me happy? . . . How can I find fulfillment in my work?*

Just as we spend one-third of our lives sleeping, another third is devoted to making a living, and it's very clear that the positive or negative qualities of those two endeavors have a vital influence on one another. But I'm not suggesting that, in order to sleep well every night, you should immediately quit your job if you don't like it. Any type of work can be made more fulfilling if it's done with simplicity and present-moment awareness.

In order to understand how this can be done, you need first to understand a very important point about the way Ayurveda approaches disease and health. Disease is viewed as actually having no reality in and of itself. The relationship between disease and health is like the relationship between darkness and light. Health is not the absence of disease; disease is the absence of health.

The Ayurvedic focus on health as a positive, active quality is such that, in some sense, Ayurveda doesn't deal with the treatment of disease at all. A disease is recognized as an area of physiology that is simply lacking in the basic concept we call health, the way a room is dark until a light is turned on. Health means wholeness, and when health is brought to a level of perfection it results in a state of complete fulfillment.

If dissatisfaction with work is affecting your health and ruining your sleep, it's not really your job that's the problem, it's the quality of your life in every area. There's an old Ayurvedic saying: "The world is as we are." Have you ever noticed how, on days when you are feeling well rested and happy, everything goes well and people respond to you quite positively? And have you noticed that on days when you feel groggy and grouchy, the world responds in that way also?

If you're rested, if you're fulfilled in other parts of your life, your work will be much more enjoyable, more efficient, and certainly more fulfilling. Although sometimes you may feel like a victim of circumstance, you actually can take charge of the situation, and the first step lies on the level of your consciousness. You don't have to go anywhere or to anyone to find fulfillment; it is inherently within you to begin with. You just have to give yourself access to that field of pure intelligence.

The first step is to make a slight shift in your awareness. It's a shift in the direction of self-indulgence in a good sense, of attention to yourself and to your purpose in life. Once you see that there's a perspective that's bigger than your worries, bigger than your professional concerns, then you'll be able to do your work much more efficiently and with much more happiness.

You'll be more focused in your work because you'll have a larger view of what it means to have a life of fulfillment and satisfaction.

BALANCE AND BEAUTY

Our lives, like the universe as a whole, should be a balance of rest and activity. Whatever decisions you make regarding your career, be sure you have time for other important things in life, like enjoying your children or grandchildren or other members of your family. These simple joys of life are an extremely important part of the Ayurvedic routine.

Don't neglect time for leisure activities, hobbies, or educational or cultural interests. There are many things that you may have been wanting to do for your whole life, but putting off because of lack of time—and this violates the principle of balancing rest and activity.

For most people who have insomnia, the activity portion of life is being overly emphasized at the expense of the rest phase. Be sure to take enough time to balance your successful, dynamic activity with genuine recreation. Don't suffer from picnic deficiency!

Free time and vacation time should be spent in activities that make you feel more whole and refreshed, not more fatigued and tired. This is a recreational universe made for those who want to share in God's one great passion: beauty. In the presence of beauty, the connection with nature is restored and we recognize it as truth.

In Ayurveda, all problems arise because of object-referral. Object-referral simply means that we refer to objects in order to identify ourselves, in order to tell ourselves who we are. These objects can be situations, circumstances, people, or things. As a result of object-referral, we develop guilts and regrets about the past, we are distracted in the present, and we experience fear and anxiety about the future. And this is the root cause of illness.

So the solution to any illness is to become self-referring. You give to the world your greatest gift when you're being yourself. Anything else causes a lot of strain, stress, fatigue, anxiety, and insomnia. The cause of suffering is the loss of the self to the self-image, the forsaking of a self-referring inner reality for an object-referring image.

In order to get back to the self, we have to learn to transcend; we have to learn to trust ourselves, our instincts, and our intuitive senses. The goal of Ayurveda is for us to realize that we are made of pure awareness, that it is our destiny to be always experiencing this fact, that it is our destiny to become free.

PRESENT-MOMENT AWARENESS

In order to experience freedom, we must have present-moment, life-centered awareness, where love and trust are naturally felt. The opposite of present-moment awareness is time-bound awareness, and the emotion that naturally accompanies it is fear.

There's a great saying by the poet Rumi: "Come out of the circle of time into the circle of love." The best way to prepare for any future event is to be fully in your present moment now. The only goal of life, therefore, for a free person, should be to allow the flow of pure awareness, the flow of relaxed attention, into the physiology so he or she can experience in crystal clarity things as they actually are, and not filtered through the camouflage of preconceived notions, definitions, interpretations, and judgments.

In this pure awareness, we see the world as it really is, a manifestation and an unfoldment of the eternal presence of the self. A person in this state of awareness is truly free, and can have the support of everything that he or she desires. In this state of awareness, wishes, dreams, desires, and commands unfold like seeds left in the ground, waiting for the appropriate season to bloom spontaneously into flowers and beautiful gardens.

Our life experiences are a result of where our attention takes us. In fact, we are the quality of our attention. If our attention is fragmented, we feel fragmented, we are fragmented. When our attention is in the past, we are in the past. When our attention is in the future, we too are in the realm of an imaginary future. But when our attention is in the present, we are in the presence of life energy. And all problems, particularly insomnia, are a diversion of our attention from present-moment awareness into time-bound awareness.

Present-moment awareness is allowing the flow of attention, the flow of consciousness, the flow of universal intelligence, the flow of nature, to move spontaneously and effortlessly through our physiologies. And when we shift our attention from object-referral to self-referral, our physiology will function with the vibrancy of life energy.

Now it turns out that being an object of self-referral instead of object-referral is actually the simplest thing we can do. It's so simple because to be one's self is our very nature. There is nothing more intimate than yourself. It is only because we have become so used to complications that it could seem difficult to be ourselves. But starting on the path of self-referral is the most natural, effortless, and enjoyable thing that anyone could ever do.

In the course of discovering ourselves, we discover our intimate connection to nature, and that this connection can never be broken. To be self-referring means to be in tune with our individual nature and with nature as a whole. This is the real path, and the only path, to perfect health.

It is very interesting that the Ayurvedic word for "health" is *swastia,* which literally means to be established in the self. So even in the very word itself we see this profound truth, that the basis of perfect health, which of course includes freedom from insomnia, is to be in touch with yourself.

Where do we find this self? It is found in the simplest form of our own awareness, of our own consciousness, where it is experienced as truly unbounded, free from limitations, completely integrated and in harmony with nature. From this level all choices we make are most natural and life-supporting. From this level we act spontaneously, intuitively, and in such a way as to promote balance and health.

IN CLOSING

In closing, let's review the major principles for dealing with insomnia.

I've emphasized the importance of achieving harmony with the cycles of nature and creating a healthy, balanced daily routine. Specifically, this means going to bed and getting up early and at the same time every day.

Remember that in order to achieve this we fix our waking time, initially using an alarm, and arising at that time no matter how we feel. If you are used to sleeping late, you can gradually move to an earlier wake-up time as described in chapter 4, and this will help you to move your bedtime earlier in a corresponding way. Achieving this natural balance in bedtime and waking time is one of the most important recommendations in this book.

If you feel restless after getting into bed and cannot fall asleep, remember to use the body-awareness techniques described in chapter 2. By using these techniques, and by maintaining an earlier bedtime and awakening time, you will begin to enjoy normalized sleep patterns and more restful sleep.

Because the state of balance of the mind is so important in achieving good sleep, let me emphasize again the value of the meditation technique—of being aware of your breath—that was introduced in chapter 6. This is the most efficient method for directly contacting your inner self and reestablishing balance in the mind. Once that balance has been achieved, it will become easy and quite natural to put into effect all of the other health-promoting recommendations of this book, such as creating harmony in the senses (as described in chapter 6).

As you bring about all these changes, always be easy on yourself. Remember that some of the recommendations are bound to work better or have a more immediate effect than others. If at first any of the suggestions seem overwhelming, then just begin by adding the ones you can easily do, and meanwhile keep reviewing the contents of the book so that, over time, you can incorporate more. Keep in mind that these recommendations are not arbitrary but simply represent the laws of nature that have to do with good sleep and good health, and with how to live your life as a whole.

One last recommendation in this regard: When we seem to fall out of balance with nature, Ayurveda says it's not that we actually lose our connection with nature; rather, it's more like we forget it. We stop recognizing a reality that is always there. So the process of regaining balance, of reestablishing self-referral, is really a process of remembering. In Ayurveda, this is called regaining *smriti,* or memory of your own nature.

The process of growth is ongoing. By gradually adding Ayurvedic elements to your personal routine, you'll find that conquering your sleep problems will be the least of your accomplishments. You'll find your life becoming increasingly natural, harmonious, and simple.

That's the ultimate purpose of everything in this book: to help you create simplicity in the mind/body system, to bring the system back into accord with nature, and to point you in the direction of self-referral. By promoting self-referral, my intention is to bring you to a higher level of self-fulfillment, which is ultimately the best way and the only real way of dealing with the problem of insomnia. You'll be more in touch with yourself, more in tune with the laws of nature, and the result of this growth will be complete fulfillment, total balance, and perfect health.

BIBLIOGRAPHY

Brody, Jane. *The New York Times,* "Personal Health" column (1/19/94 and 1/26/94).

Dement, Dr. William C. *The Sleepwatchers* (Stanford, Calif.: Portable Stanford Book Series, 1992).

Ford, Norman. *Good Night* (Rockport, Mass.: Para Research, 1983).

Hauri, Peter, and Shirley Linde. *No More Sleepless Nights* (New York: John Wiley & Sons, 1990).

Regenstein, Dr. Quentin, and David Ritchie. *Sleep Problems and Solutions* (Mount Vernon, N.Y.: Consumer Reports Books, 1990).

Schlereth, Thomas J. *Victorian America* (New York: Harper Perennial, 1992).

Sweeney, Dr. Donald R. *Overcoming Insomnia* (New York: G. P. Putnam's Sons, 1989).

Sources

More information on Mind/Body and Ayurvedic treatments, products, herbs, and educational programs can be obtained from the following organizations:

Quantum Publications
P.O. Box 598
South Lancaster, MA 01561
800-858-1808

Quantum Publications, Inc., is a Massachusetts corporation beneficially owned by Dr. Deepak Chopra and his family.

The Chopra Center for Well-Being
7630 Fay Avenue
La Jolla, CA 92037
1-888-424-6772 (toll-free)
619-551-7788

Ayurvedic Institute
1311 Menaul N.E., Suite A
Albuquerque, NM 87112
505-291-9698

American Institute of Vedic Studies
P.O. Box 8357
Santa Fe, NM 87504

American School of Ayurvedic Sciences
10025 N.E. 4th Street
Bellevue, WA 98004
206-453-8022

Maharishi Ayurved Products
P.O. Box 541
Lancaster, MA 01523
800-255-8332

Shivani Ayurvedic Personal Care Products
P.O. Box 377
Lancaster, MA 01523
800-237-8221

Auromere Ayurvedic Imports
1291 Weber St.
Pomona, CA 91768
909-629-0108

Deepak Chopra and Infinite Possibilities International offer a
wide range of seminars, products, and educational programs.
For additional information, please contact: Infinite Possibilities
International, 60 Union Avenue, Sudbury, MA 01778, U.S.A.,
1-800-858-1808 (toll-free)/508-440-8400. For medical in-
quiries and health-related programs, please contact: The
Chopra Center for Well-Being, 7630 Fay Avenue, La Jolla, CA
92037, U.S.A., 1-888-424-6772 (toll-free)/619-551-7788.

INDEX